DID YOU KNOW . . . ?

- White bread is high in fiber and contains *more* calcium than whole-grain breads?

- French Fries are high in Vitamin C, fiber and potassium—and, when well cooked, contain little saturated fat?

- The good old American hamburger—knocked around by diet books these days—is a goldmine of protein, iron and B vitamins—and the bun offers all the same low-fat goodies found in white bread?

- Cereal "health" bars, once a good idea, now contain high levels of added sugar, salt, and vegetable fat—often of the saturated kind?

- "Fresh" fruit which has been sitting for days on your supermarket shelf may have lost some of its vitamins and freshness—and may have even been irradiated or chemically treated?

NOW YOU'LL KNOW, with the diet you thought you could only dream about, just how satisfying *and* effective losing weight can be. Judith Wills, an internationally known diet expert and researcher, has been an editor of the popular diet magazine *Slimmer* for years. She has built a strong reputation for giving sensible advice that really works. N methods that have worked of others who have lost we

THE ⌷
FOOD DIET

THE
JUNK
FOOD
DIET

Judith Wills

ST. MARTIN'S PRESS/NEW YORK

The Junk Food Diet was previously published by The Penguin Group in Great Britain, in a somewhat altered form.

THE JUNK FOOD DIET

ISBN: 0-312-92182-9

Printed in the United States of America

First St. Martin's Press mass market edition/March 1990

10 9 8 7 6 5 4 3 2 1

❖ Note to Readers ❖

❖ Contents ❖

Defining "junk" food . . . how the "healthy
eating" movement has done harm as well as
good . . . why there's no such thing as an
"unhealthy" food . . . examples of "healthy
junk" and "junky health" foods . . . why you
shouldn't feel guilty for eating foods you like
. . . how you can lose weight *and* stay within
the United States Department of Agriculture
Dietary Guidelines for Healthy Americans
eating guidelines on "junk" food . . . the
benefits and principles of The Junk Food Diet.

How healthy-eating myths arise . . . the
pitfalls of the healthy-eating mania . . . what
our bodies really need for good health . . .
dietary guidelines and eating recommendations
. . . why there's no need to give up red meat
or dairy products . . . sugar and your health
. . . coping with a sweet tooth . . . the truth
about salt in your diet . . . the fiber debate—
fiber chart . . . vitamin C charts, calcium
charts . . . vitamins and minerals and junk-

don't need to follow a low-calorie diet for life
. . . why you shouldn't compare your food
intake with anyone else's . . . how to build
up your calorie level gradually . . . your
maintenance diet . . . eating and life-style
tips . . . what to do should the unthinkable
happen! . . . learning to be a thin person . . .
three simple stages to beat binges forever.

How kids' nutrition needs differ from adults'
. . . how many of the foods kids love are good
for them! . . . why there is no need to ban
sweet foods from your child's diet . . . the
simple traffic-light guide to a healthy "junk"
diet for your child . . . junk food and the
additives debate . . . overweight children—
how to slim them down painlessly . . .
height/weight graphs for kids . . . planning
your child's menu.

How to use the recipe section . . . succulent
sauces . . . super bread snacks . . . tasty egg
and cheese meals . . . unboring fish meals
. . . chicken and turkey dishes . . . pasta and
rice dishes . . . red-meat dishes galore.

❖ Introduction ❖

JUNK FOOD IS FATTENING FOOD.

If you really want to lose weight, you'll have to alter your diet radically.

The only way to lose weight is to become a vegetarian.

These are just some of the phrases you've been hearing—until you're sick of them—over the past few years.

Now I'm blatantly and guiltlessly going to lead you into rebellion! Stick with me and I'll show you how you can lose, and stay healthy, on all the food you like—without ever having to eat cottage cheese again!

It was perhaps inevitable that the diet industry would jump on the healthy-eating bandwagon. What makes a healthy diet has been one of the big talking points of the 1980s. Guided by various trials and studies, culminating in the 1989 National Research Council's Diet and Health Report—whose main suggestion was that we should reduce our consumption of fat—self-appointed diet gurus have virtually led us to believe that all foods containing animal fat—or, by the way, sugar, salt, or additives, or without a large dose of bran—are akin to arsenic, and that to eat them and, heaven forbid, enjoy them is a sin!

Most of the famous diet books of the 1980s have gone along with these ideas, recommending diets very low in (or free from) meat, high in raw foods, vegetables, and fruit, packed full of fiber and vigorously avoiding anything processed.

Yes, the health-food lobby has helped us greatly in leading us to a more enlightened, balanced way of eating. But I am sure that a grossly limited diet is not the way to good health—or permanent weight loss. There are millions of people in the Western world who have tried these "new health"-style diets and failed, long term, to lose weight on them, or, indeed, to become "healthier."

Were you one of them?

No wonder you couldn't follow the high-fruit diet for long. It upset your stomach and made you light-headed. No wonder you didn't like the high-fiber diet. You couldn't put up with the gas and the bloating. No wonder you lost weight on the liquids-only diet, but put it all back on within weeks. It didn't help your day-to-day eating habits.

Limited-eating fad diets are definitely not what weight loss for life is all about. And they are not what you want.

What the famous weight-loss gurus forgot was that you can't change a nation's diet drastically and expect us all to adapt. It can't work for more than a while. That's why lost weight returns within a year for many dieters.

The foods you've been raised on must form a large part of any successful diet: meat, cheese, eggs, potatoes, bread. And so must all the foods that have, in the last twenty years or so, become an important part of our lives: the takeouts, the pizzas, the burgers, the fried chicken.

These are all foods that have, in recent years, been saddled with the label "junk." They are the foods that we are now made to feel guilty about eating and enjoying.

And yet sales figures and my own surveys prove that these are the foods you like (even if they are no longer the foods you have the nerve to serve when guests come to dinner).

So, for a change, I've got some good news for you. I'm going to show you just why so-called "junk" food isn't junk food at all, and that there is no such thing as a "healthy" food—or, for that matter, an "unhealthy" one.

And I'm going to tell you how you can lose weight —and stay thin for life—on the food you really like.

Burgers, hot dogs, frozen dinners, potato chips, french fries, baked potatoes, mashed potatoes, white bread, burritos, nachos, Chinese takeout, pizza, bacon, fish, chili, spaghetti, fried chicken, fried fish, manicotti, cannoli.

Are you beginning to like the sound of this? I haven't finished! You can also lose weight—and stay thin—without having to give up the treats you like best: chocolate, ice cream, cookies, cakes, desserts, cheesecake, even alcohol; in fact, all the things you thought you could never eat on a reducing diet—let alone a healthy one!

What's more, I'm going to tell you how you need not—unless you want to—eat vegetarian meals, grapefruit, cottage cheese, farmer's cheese, brown rice, steamed fish, Melba toast, celery, carrot sticks, or lettuce ever again!

On my Junk Food Diet you will lose weight easily

because you won't feel deprived of your favorite foods—or anxious that you've got to grapple with a whole new style of eating. You needn't worry about how the family will react to different menus or, alternatively, have to bother with cooking separate meals for yourself. Everyone can follow this diet, whether or not he or she is trying to lose weight.

You need spend no extra money or go hunting for unusual ingredients. You need not go near health-food stores or attempt to master vegetarian cookery. I'm going to show you how you can continue to shop at your favorite supermarket or local grocery store. And—most important—you needn't worry or feel guilty that in some way you are damaging your health by eating the foods you like.

The Junk Food Diet will show you how so-called "junk foods" and "everyday foods" can be part of your regular eating pattern and still give you a diet well within those United States Department of Agriculture Dietary Guidelines (given in detail in Chapter 2).

The Junk Food Diet doesn't expect you to attempt the impossible. It does expect you to want to carry on with your normal life.

So, if you desperately want to get thin and yet still be able to say yes to the supermarket, yes to family food, yes to takeout, yes to frozen dinners, yes to cans and packages and jars, then here is your diet.

It's all you need to stay thin—and healthy—for life.

❖ 1. ❖

The Case
for
Junk Food

EVERY ONE OF US KNOWS A "HEALTH FREAK" WHO piously raises an eyebrow at the sight of our digging into french fries or a steak or—heaven forbid—sliced white bread with real butter on it. "How can you eat that junk?" the health-food fanatic will say.

Yet, what is junk?

Long before burgers were invented "junk" was the dry, salted meat that sailors ate on board ship when it was a choice between that or starvation. In the sixties and seventies junk became another word for fast food and sweet snacks. But today the word *junk* has been used with greater and greater abandon. Some dictionaries describe it as "food of poor nutritional quality" or "food of little nutritional value." These phrases are, of necessity, vague, because in the precise world of applied nutrition there is no such thing as "junk food"! And when I began asking around for ordinary people's definition of junk, I began to understand why dieticians don't use the word.

In my verbal poll I asked a wide cross-section of people from all incomes and age groups to say exactly what they would classify as junk food. The foods mentioned most often were these: sugary foods, chocolate, sweets, french fries, fast food, store-bought cakes, cookies, soda, and powdered drink mixes.

Not far behind were these: ice cream, red meat, Cheddar cheese, pasta, white bread, white rice, cornflakes and other cereals, and canned fruit.

By this time I was beginning to feel surprised that so many people felt so many foods were junk. And as my questioning progressed, I became more and more surprised. Here are some other answers I got to the question "What is your definition of junk food?": all packaged foods, all canned foods, all processed foods, all foods containing added sugar, all foods containing added salt, all foods containing additives of any kind, all foods with some of their natural fiber content removed.

There's more. A few people even said: all cooked food, all food that has been altered in any way from its natural state.

I finished my little survey and looked at my lists. I got out my nutrition books and spent a long time searching for foods not on my list of "junk." Do you know what I ended up with? The only foods that no one mentioned at all as being junk were: fresh fruit; fresh, raw vegetables; fresh herbs; naturally dried nuts, seeds, grains, and beans; and wild birds and game (tracked and killed yourself, of course). That was all that was left.

My survey proved what I have suspected—that although the "healthy eating" movement of the last decade has undoubtedly done us in the Western world a great deal of good, it has also done us harm. It has made us feel guilty about enjoying a wide variety of foods that are certainly not of "little nutritional value." It has made us fearful of damaging our health by eating almost anything from bread to bacon. If we listen to the anti-junk-food doom-sayers' advice and cut out most of the things we enjoy, I believe we will limit our diets to such an extent that for every twentieth-century ill we prevent, we'll cause a new one. Let's return to that oh-so-short list of "non-junk foods." Far from making up the perfect, healthy diet, they present certain problems.

First, it would be very difficult to eat a healthy diet—one containing all the nutrients we need, long-term—from such a limited selection of foods. So many of us would become ill through deficiency diseases.

Then, few of us could stick to such a diet for long in any case. Think about it. Could you live on raw fruit and vegetables, feed a family, socialize, travel, work, and live happily on those foods—even for a few days? No. Neither could I. I wouldn't want to. And we don't have to.

The idea that only a chosen few foods aren't junk is plainly ridiculous. And it is a terrible shame that we have to feel guilty about eating the things we like best.

These conclusions are backed up by the government's National Food Consumption Survey and sales figures for foods such as french fries, chocolate, and takeout.

It is nonsense to suggest that all processed and packaged food is junk, nonsense to say that all food containing saturated fat, or salt, or sugar is junk, and nonsense for the health-food faddists to expect us to give them up.

HEALTHY JUNK FOOD

Let's take a closer look at some of the foods most frequently described as "junk" and see what's really in them.

Takeout

Takeout can mean anything from chop suey to cheeseburgers, so it's impossible to lump them all together in one nutritional bag. At worst they can be high in fat and salt, and low in fiber and vitamins. But at best they can be—and often are—of good nutritional value.

White bread

My junk-food-poll participants said white bread is junk because "it has no fiber and no goodness left in it." In fact, white bread does still contain fiber. It also contains protein and iron, and, unlike wholemeal bread, it is often fortified with vitamins and minerals. What's more, it has slightly less fat than whole wheat.

Cheddar (and other hard) cheese

Frowned upon because "it's full of animal fat," cheese is a good source of protein and is one of our major sources of calcium—unlike the soft cheeses, such as cottage cheese.

French fries

"Nothing good in them," "full of saturated fat." In fact, well-cooked fries fried in corn oil still have lots of vitamin C, have a reasonable amount of fiber, and have a lot of potassium. They contain little saturated fat.

Hamburgers

"Red meat is bad for you." The average grilled or broiled fried and drained burger is a good source of protein, iron, and B vitamins, plus, in the bun, all the same goodness you get in white bread.

Tacos

"Loaded with fat" is the usual cry. Actually, when made with ground beef, lots of lettuce and tomato, it's one of the healthiest meals around. A little known fact—taco shells are a surprisingly good source of calcium.

Eggs and bacon

"My wife forbids me to eat it because of all the fat." What a shame. Trimmed bacon, grilled or fried until crisp, with a fried egg, both drained on paper towels, has B vitamins, iron, lots of protein, and surprisingly little fat. It's a meal that will set any husband (or wife) up for the day!

Are you feeling less guilty yet? All the preceding foods (and hundreds more like them) are far from being junk; they are high in "nutritional value."

And if you like them, you'd be silly to banish them from your diet.

HEALTH FOOD—BUT IS IT?

In just the same way that "junk" foods are often condemned without a fair trial, many foods are now being sold as "health" foods when, in fact, they are no more healthy than the foods we eat as junk.

Following are just some of the so-called "health foods" that may not be as healthy as they seem.

Granola

"The healthiest breakfast you can eat," said several people when I delved into their views on a healthy diet. "High in fiber and full of natural goodness," said someone else. And so original Swiss muesli, on which granola is based, was—yet many brands of granola contain sugar as one of the prime ingredients. Ah, but brown sugar. That's no better for you than white. Just as many granolas also contain lots of added salt. And to make matters worse, granola is no higher in fiber than many other low-health-profile breakfast cereals! Worst of all, it's *loaded* with fat.

Cereal bars and "health" bars

"Much better for you than a chocolate or candy bar." Perhaps the original concept of high-fiber cereal bars was good, but nearly all now contain high levels of sugar or one of its close relatives, fructose and glucose. They also contain salt and vegetable fat (often of the saturated kind). I bought a carob-coated "health" bar and the list of ingredients read: sugar, palm kernel and palm oil (saturated), skim-milk powder, lingoes, carob powder, maltodextrin (a form of carbohydrate), lecithin (an emulsifier), and salt.

Whole-grain bread

"Much better for you than white." Whole-meal bread's "plus" is that it contains more fiber than ordinary white bread. It has only slightly more fiber than white bread and often contains more fat.

Honey

"Natural sweetness." Natural sweetness is just another word for sugar, and there's precious little else in honey.

Fruit

"Fresh, natural, full of vitamins." This is an extreme example, I know, and of course good-quality fresh fruit can't be called "junk." But go into any supermarket at the wrong time of the week or the wrong week of the year and you are liable to end up with a piece of fruit that is neither fresh nor full of vitamins. Fruit stored too long, especially in warm, light conditions, like under a shop awning in summer, will have lost a lot, or even most, of its vitamin C before you eat it. Natural? How do you know it hasn't been sprayed with a variety of chemicals for pest and disease control?

* * *

So, you see, things aren't always what they seem. In Chapter 2 I'll be looking more closely at all the nutrients we need for good health, and discussing how The Junk Food Diet provides them for you within U.S.D.A. dietary guidelines.

But what I want you to begin to realize is that you don't have to feel guilty about liking burgers, burritos, Chinese takeout, fries, and hot dogs. You don't have to pretend to your friends, like a closet eater, that you don't eat these things.

No food properly prepared and eaten within a varied diet is junk. Individual foods are not "healthy" or "unhealthy." It is how those foods join together to make up your diet over the weeks that will decide whether you're as healthy through nutrition as you could be.

So, although there are no junk foods, there *is* a junk diet—an unbalanced, limited diet within which you're getting too much of certain nutrients and too few of others. What you don't want to do is eat one or two foods to the exclusion of most others, whether your favorite happens to be ice cream and milk shakes—or oranges. You can end up with a junk diet just as easily through eating too many of the so-called "healthy" foods as you can on chocolate and chips. For instance, let's imagine you decide to go on a "health kick" and eat nothing but oranges. You'd very soon get bad stomachaches, and would have to spend most of your day in the bathroom. If you stayed on the diet for many weeks you might get diseases like anemia and rickets.

Of course, you wouldn't be so silly, but the fact is that fad eating of any kind will eventually make you unhealthy, and will often make you fat.

So eat your favorite foods within a varied diet. Eat your fries twice a week or maybe even more often. Eat a chocolate bar or a couple of oranges every day, if that's what you really like. There is plenty of room in your diet for all the foods you love.

And don't worry—you don't need to be weighed down with a nutrition textbook. The Junk Food Diet will show you how to eat, and get thin on your favorite foods—for life.

HOW JUNK FOODS CAN HELP YOU LOSE WEIGHT

Okay, so now you're convinced that you can join me on this rebellious diet without ruining your health. But can you really lose weight on all those fattening foods you love?

Yes, you can!

Let's look at what you have to do to lose weight:

Fact one: You can't lose weight unless, over a period of time, you take in (in what you eat and drink) fewer calories than your body will use up in its normal energy requirements. If your body isn't getting the energy it needs from the food and drink you put into it, it will get energy instead from the stored fat supplies within your body. So—like magic—you will get thinner!

Fact two: There is no method of losing weight (apart from temporary fluid weight) that will really work apart from the above method. You can help the fat-burning process along by stepping up your exercise levels so you use more energy (see Chapter 5).

Fact three: The number of calories you can eat

and still lose weight varies enormously. A normal daily calorie consumption for a woman of average weight and height to maintain her weight is around 2,000. For a man of average weight and height the figure is around 2,700. If you are overweight, you have probably been eating more than that amount. It doesn't have to be a lot more. In calorie terms, one pound of fat on your body equals 3,500 calories you ate or drank that you didn't need. So, for example, if you are a woman and you eat 2,500 calories a day when you really need only 2,000 a day, within one week—only seven days—you will have eaten 3,500 (2,500 − 2,000 × 7) calories more than you need and you may have put on one pound in weight!

That extra 500 calories a day represents one small snack. So don't think you have to be a pig to get fat. You don't. Now, let's look at it the other way. You want to lose weight because you've been eating a steady 2,500 calories a day and it's made you fat. If you drop down to 1,500 calories a day (far more than most low-calorie diets suggest), you will be giving yourself a daily calorie deficit of 1,000. Over a week that is 7,000 calories. To lose a pound of fat you have to have a deficit of 3,500 calories, so eating as much as 1,500 calories a day, you'll lose two pounds a week. That's 104 pounds in a year. Enough for almost anyone, I'd guess!

Of course, there are some people who for various reasons will need to diet on less than 1,500 calories a day. Some lucky people (mostly men) will be able to diet on more than 1,500 calories a day. All I want to point out here is that you won't be going hungry on The Junk Food Diet, and once your calorie level for dieting is decided upon (which it will be in Chapter 6), you will still lose whether you eat your calorie allowance in pizza or in celery, in apple pie or in cottage cheese.

No matter what you have read in any previous diet, there is no special food that will make you lose weight. The only way to lose is to reduce your calorie intake. And I'm going to show you how you can cut those calories down to the right level for you within your eating preferences. No drastic alterations in what you eat. I'm going to show how you can turn a "fattening" diet—the kind you've been eating up until now—into a weight-loss diet, and a healthy one.

Following are some actual examples of high-calorie diets turned, quite easily, into low-calorie, healthy ones.

Example One

Susan, an average, active eighteen-year-old, weighs 154 pounds. At 5 feet, 6 inches tall, she is 21 pounds overweight. Her weight gain began in grade school, but has become worse in the last year since she started college and began living away from home.

"I won't eat anything for breakfast except toast. I always have lunch in the college cafeterias, where choice is limited, and in the evening I like a takeout meal because I can't stand cooking. I've no real food favorites, though—I'm easy to please as long as things are quick and easy."

Here's what Susan ate in a typical day:

Breakfast

2 slices toast from large loaf, liber-
ally spread with butter and jam   440 calories

Mid-morning snack
1 plain croissant   235 calories

Lunch
1 cheese enchilada, guacamole,
  and salad   675 calories

Mid-afternoon snack
1 small packet peanuts (2 ounces;
  55 grams)   275 calories

Dinner
1 7-inch cheese-and-onion pizza   340 calories
tossed salad with dressing   145 calories
1 apple   125 calories
1 glass red wine   75 calories

Late evening
1 large slice bread, liberally
  spread with butter   165 calories

Throughout day
5 cups coffee with cream and
  sugar   265 calories
                    Total   2,740 calories

This total is probably around 500 calories a day
more than Susan should be eating, and it accounts
for her steady weight increase. With minor changes
to her diet, and no hunger, she can reduce the total
to around 1,500 a day for a good weekly weight loss.
The new-look day's eating (right) also matches up
well with nutrition guidelines (see Table 2, page 30)
as it gives 62 grams protein, 880 milligrams cal-

cium, 45 grams fat (equivalent to just under 30 percent of her day's energy intake), 25 grams (minimum) fiber, 11.5 grams+ iron, approximately 45 milligrams vitamin C. Three grams of sodium is well below the recommended 6-gram limit.

THE CASE FOR JUNK FOOD

Breakfast
2 slices toast from thinly cut loaf, lightly spread with 2 teaspoons butter and 2 teaspoons reduced-sugar jelly	150 calories

Mid-morning snack
1 hard roll with 2 teaspoons reduced-calorie jam	170 calories

Lunch
1 Wendy's taco salad	390 calories

Mid-afternoon snack
1-ounce bag nacho tortilla chips	150 calories

Dinner
2 slices cheese and onion pizza	340 calories
salad with low-calorie Italian dressing	20 calories
1 small apple	80 calories
1 glass red wine	75 calories

Late evening
1 thin slice bread, lightly spread with butter	85 calories

Throughout day
5 cups coffee with skim milk and
    artificial sweetener   <u>70 calories</u>
                                Total   1,530 calories

Example Two

Mary, a thirty-eight-year-old mother of two pre-
teen children, has a part-time morning job. She's 5
feet, 2 inches tall and weighs 147 pounds. Before she
had children she weighed 119 pounds. Lately she's
been trying to diet, without success, by cutting out
between-meal snacks. "Also, although I'm not very
hungry at breakfast time, I've been trying to eat a
good breakfast to 'set me up' for the day. Even so,
I'm very hungry when I get home at lunchtime."

Mary has to cook an evening meal for the family
at 6 P.M. "So I'm always hungry again by ten, but I
make do with a milk drink before bed."

Here's what Mary ate in a typical day:

Breakfast
average bowlful (2½ ounces) gra-
    nola
½ cup milk   380 calories
1 medium slice toast with butter
    and honey   120 calories

Lunch
2-egg omelet cooked in butter,
    with large helping of french
    fries and ½ cup peas   740 calories
1 frozen yogurt   180 calories

Dinner

1 serving homemade lasagna	480 calories
Italian garlic bread	205 calories
salad with Italian dressing	100 calories

Late evening

cocoa and two peanut-butter cookies		<u>220 calories</u>
	Total	2,425 calories

Mary has been gaining weight on this diet because, as she isn't very tall, she probably needs only 2,000 calories a day. Although Mary believes she is doing her best to diet, she is making several mistakes. There's no point in having a big breakfast if you don't really want one. Cutting out snacks doesn't work if you simply eat more calories at your regular meals. And she's wasting calories on lots of very high-fat items, when lower-fat ones would do just as well. Granola, by the way, is a deceptive food: it is heavy in weight, and even a small bowlful is high in calories.

Here's a new-look day that should result in easy weight loss for Mary.

Breakfast

2 shredded-wheat biscuits (1 ounce) with 3/4 cup 2% low-fat milk	195 calories

Mid-morning

1 medium slice bread with low-fat spread and honey (taken to work)	145 calories

Lunch
2-egg omelet with mushrooms,
  green peppers, and onions
  cooked without butter; semi-
  small order french fries; 1 cup
  peas   490 calories

Dinner
1 serving homemade lasagna, using Junk Food Diet method (see
  recipe, page 282)   350 calories
1/2 cup carrots, boiled
salad with low-calorie Italian
  dressing   30 calories
1 cup strawberries   45 calories

Suppertime snack
1 medium slice toast with diet
  margarine   70 calories
1 Carnation 70-calorie rich choco-
  late drink   70 calories
                          Total   1,400 calories

Mary's new diet is also sound nutritionally, as she gets 67 grams of protein, 650 milligrams of calcium, 45 grams of fat (equivalent to 29 percent of her day's energy intake), 26 grams of fiber, 11 milligrams of iron, approximately 60 milligrams of vitamin C, approximately 2,380 milligrams of sodium.

Example Three
  Twenty-three-year-old Jack works as a delivery-man for a city furniture store. He is 5 feet, 9 inches tall, weighs 168 pounds, and would like to lose about

15 pounds. He shares an apartment with other men. Living a typical bachelor existence, he snatches food when and where he can, and he eats lots of takeout meals. Evenings are often spent at his favorite watering hole.

"I feel that my diet is unhealthy but I don't know what to do. I can't sit around eating cottage cheese and raw vegetables. My co-workers and roommates would laugh at me."

Here's what Jack ate in a typical day:

Breakfast
2 shredded-wheat biscuits with 1
   cup milk   250 calories

Mid-morning snack
1 McDonald's Quarterpounder
   with cheese   525 calories
1 large cola   143 calories

Afternoon snack
Snickers Bar   290 calories

Evening snack
ham-and-cheese sandwich   355 calories
                                           approx.

Drinks
4 bottles beer   600 calories

Evening meal
Long John Silver's three-piece fish
   dinner   940 calories

Throughout day
4 to 5 cups of coffee with milk, no
   sugar   150 calories
                Total   3,430 calories

A new-look day for Jack means he can still have
several snacks and meals, and visit the bar, but the
calories are greatly reduced. With a little fruit
added, he now has a diet well within the U.S.D.A.
guidelines at 107 grams of protein, 56 grams of fat,
(25 percent of the day's energy total), 25 grams of
fiber, 10 milligrams of iron, 84 milligrams of vitamin C, 900 milligrams of calcium, and the sodium is
kept to 2,500 milligrams.

Breakfast
2 shredded-wheat biscuits with 1
   cup skim milk   190 calories
1 small orange   55 calories

Mid-morning snack
1-ounce package potato chips   150 calories

Lunch
1 McDonald's Quarterpounder (no
   cheese)
diet cola
1 piece fresh fruit (taken to work)   550 calories

Afternoon snack
1 Twix   140 calories

Light meal (7 P.M.—bought from freezer case on
   way home)

1 Green Giant Beef Burgundy
  with Rice
1 cup frozen peas   330 calories

Drinks
2 bottles beer   300 calories

Evening meal
1 Long John Silver's Baked Fish
  with Sauce   150 calories
1 ear of corn   100 calories

Throughout day
1 cup of milk for coffee (milk at
  home is skim, but whole milk
  used during day)   100 calories
                           Total   2,100 calories

So here you have the proof that it isn't difficult to
cut down on calories while still eating plenty, and
still eating the way you like! And by following The
Junk Food Diet, you'll do just that. It lets you eat all
your favorite foods within a healthy, overall plan.

Here is a list of the many benefits of following
The Junk Food Diet:

It takes account of your own likes and dislikes.
There's plenty of choice on the first part, the Set
Diet. But when you begin the second part, the Pick
Your Own Plan, there's almost unlimited flexibility.

It's easy. There are no complicated menus, recipes or calculations. You can eat as simply as you
like.

It's familiar. There are no unusual dishes or exotic ingredients to worry about. You'll find all the meals and snacks you know.

It's convenient. You pick the way you want to eat. There are meals suitable for any situation, and there's a special "Eating out" section.

You won't go hungry. Before you begin dieting, we find the right calorie level for you, so you won't go hungry by following a diet that's too meager.

It doesn't make you enemies! Most diets don't get the approval of your family and friends. This one will, because family and friends will hardly notice you are dieting.

It doesn't deprive you. You decide what foods you really can't live without, and The Junk Food Diet says yes, you can eat them!

It's for life. When you've slimmed down to the size you want to be, I show you exactly what to do next so you don't put the weight back on—ever!

A SUMMARY OF WHAT YOU'VE READ IN CHAPTER 1

- There is no such thing as a "junk" food or a "health" food, only a good diet or a poor diet.
- A poor diet is a limited diet.
- A good diet is a varied diet.
- You can lose weight and eat healthfully on a diet that includes all your favorite foods.

✤ 2. ✤

Healthy Eating—
the Fads and the Facts

Deaths from coronary heart disease (CHD) in the U.S. have fallen since 1964; in fact, the death rate has dropped by more than 42 percent, according to the Surgeon General's Report on Nutrition and Health, published in 1988.

"Ah!" says the health-food lobby gleefully. "A perfect example of how enlightened eating can help us beat our twentieth-century diseases!"

In fact, it isn't. For the first four years that the heart-disease rate declined, fat consumption in the United States actually increased to a record level of nearly 45 percent of energy intake. And after twenty years that level is still around 37 percent—much higher than the recommended level.

By mentioning these facts I don't mean to infer that the advice the experts have given us to eat less fat is not valid. I simply point out that when it comes to the links between diet, health, and disease, evidence and opinion are often contradictory. Out of all the speculation, debate, clinical research, and field trials, very little proof of these links has actually been forthcoming.

Even when writing the U.S.D.A.'s Dietary Guidelines (see Table 1, page 29), all the evidence the panel reviewed "fell short of proof," even though the panel felt it wise to give advice on the basis that the dietary measures recommended would certainly do us no harm and would probably do at least some good.

This kind of caution doesn't go down well with people who desperately want to believe that we can cure or prevent all our ills by the foods we eat—or the foods we avoid. Health through diet is a very appealing concept as an alternative to our modern dependence on traditional medicine and surgery practices. And it is a short step from wanting something to work to believing it really does work and then to crusading for the cause. And that is how "healthy eating" myths spring up. Unproven theories become absolute facts, facts become exaggerated—by word of mouth, in print, on TV—and suddenly eating is a dangerous pastime.

The postwar concept of food as not only necessary sustenance but also as fun, enjoyment, and harmless pleasure has been virtually crushed out of existence. The years of plenty must be replaced by years of prudence; if not, we will have to take full responsibility for the consequences (namely, our own ill health). Eating today is a stressful, guilt-ridden occupation.

And yet I'm sure that the experts responsible for the dietary advice of the 1980s did not intend to have this effect. After all, guilt and stress can cause illness, too!

In fact, experts didn't say not to eat red meat. They didn't say not to eat dairy products. There was no mention of banishing sugar from your life, or abandoning salt. Even more important, we are living longer, healthier lives than ever before in the history of mankind, so we can't be doing it all wrong.

Let's stop worrying for a minute and take a sensible look at what really does constitute a healthy diet.

Much of the advice we have received in the past decade revolves around what I call "negative nutrition," telling us what not to eat. But the basis of healthy eating is, and always has been, "positive nutrition"—making sure that we get all the nutrients we need for growth, health, and body repair. These are:

Protein

The body's "building blocks" for healthy growth and maintenance of muscle, organs, tissue—the whole works. Found in animal and plant foods.

Carbohydrate

Sugars, starches and fiber. They give us the energy (calories) we need to stay alive, move and maintain body weight—the body's fuel. Found in plant foods and milk products, but not in meat or fish.

Fat

Another fuel which also provides essential fatty acids. There are three main types of fat—saturated, monounsaturated and polyunsaturated—in animal and plant foods.

Vitamins

Needed in minute quantities to help our bodies work properly.

Minerals

Again, needed in small quantities for growth and repair and to help regulate body processes.

We also need water, the major constituent of our bodies without which we would quickly die.

Most of us feed ourselves and stay in good health without ever referring to a nutrition textbook, and I'm not suggesting that you cut out this list and take it with you to the supermarket. But just to show you that there are many, many nutrients that we need and couldn't do without in the foods that we may feel guilty about eating, look at Table 2.

The National Research Council's Diet and Health Report, Implications for Reducing Chronic Disease Risk of 1989 Recommends:

1. Reduce total fat intake to 30% or less of total calorie intake.
2. Every day eat five or more servings of a combination of vegetables and fruits, especially green and yellow vegetables and citrus fruits. Also, increase intake of starches and other complex carbohydrates by eating six or more daily servings of a combination of breads, cereals, and legumes.
3. Maintain protein intake at moderate levels.
4. Balance food intake and physical activity to maintain appropriate body weight.
5. For those who drink alcoholic beverages the committee recommends limiting consumption to the

Table 1

The United States Department of Agriculture and the United States Department of Health and Human Services Recommend in the Dietary Guidelines for Americans:

1. Eat a variety of foods.
2. Maintain a desirable weight.
3. Avoid too much fat, saturated fat, and cholesterol.
4. Eat foods with adequate starch and fiber.
5. Avoid too much sugar.
6. Avoid too much sodium.
7. If you drink alcoholic beverages, do so in moderation.

equivalent of less than 1 ounce of pure alcohol in a single day.
6. Limit total intake of sodium chloride to 6 grams or less per day.
7. Maintain adequate calcium intake.
8. Avoid taking dietary supplements in excess of the R.D.A. in any one day.
9. Maintain an optimal intake of fluoride, particularly during the years of primary and secondary tooth formation and growth.

The American Heart Association, in its Dietary Guidelines for Healthy American Adults, recommends:

1. Total fat intake should be less than 30% of total calorie intake.

2. Saturated-fat intake should be less than 10% of total calorie intake.
3. Poly-unsaturated-fat intake should not exceed 10% of total calorie intake.
4. Cholesterol intake should not exceed 300 milligrams a day.
5. Carbohydrate intake should constitute 50 percent or more of calories, with emphasis on complex carbohydrates.
6. Protein intake should provide the remainder of the calories.
7. Sodium intake should not exceed 3 grams per day.
8. Alcoholic consumption should not exceed 1 to 2 ounces of ethanol per day. Two ounces of 100-proof whiskey, 8 ounces of wine, or 24 ounces of beer each contains 1 ounce of ethanol.
9. Total calories should be sufficient to maintain the individual's recommended body weight.
10. A wide variety of foods should be consumed.

Table 2

WHAT OUR BODIES NEED FOR HEALTH

Nutrient	What it does for you
protein	builds, repairs and replaces tissue
carbohydrates	source of energy
fat	source of energy and supply of transfatty acids
fiber	for correct functioning of digestive system

Nutrient	What it does for you
iron	vital for oxygen transport around body
calcium	for formation and maintenance of bones and teeth
vitamin A	for night vision, healthy skin, and hair
vitamin B$_1$ *(thiamine)*	helps release energy from carbohydrate foods
vitamin B$_2$ *(riboflavin)*	helps release energy from protein, carbohydrates, and fat foods
vitamin B$_3$ *(niacin)*	works with thiamine and riboflavin to produce energy in the cells
vitamin B$_6$ *(pyridoxine)*	assists in absorption and metabolism of *protein;* helps body use fats
vitamin B$_{12}$	helps form red cells
folic acid	as above
vitamin C *(ascorbic acid)*	for healthy tissue and healing
vitamin D	for correct calcium utilization for formation of bones and teeth
vitamin E *(tocopherol)*	aids in formation of red blood cells and muscles

	Recommended daily amount	*Best sources*
(protein)	up to 25% of energy intake	meat, fish, poultry, dairy products

	Recommended daily amount	Best sources
(carbohydrates)	up to 55% of total energy intake	bread, potatoes, cereals, rice, beans, fruits, vegetables
(fat)	up to 30% of total energy intake	oil, butter, lard, margarine
(fiber)	25 to 30 grams	cereals, nuts, fruit, vegetables
(iron)	18 milligrams	red meat, liver, egg yolks, green leafy vegetables, dried fruits
(calcium)	1,000 milligrams	dairy products, green vegetables, sardines, canned salmon with bones
(vitamin A)	5,000 I.U.	dairy products; yellow, orange, and dark green vegetables; liver; eggs
(vitamin B_1)	1.5 milligrams	pork (especially ham),

	Recommended daily amount	Best sources
		liver, rice, bread, whole grains, pasta, peas
(vitamin B_2)	1.7 milligrams	milk, meat, cereals, eggs, whole grains, mushrooms, legumes
(vitamin B_3)	20 milligrams	meat, fish, cereals, poultry, nuts, legumes
(vitamin B_6)	2.0 milligrams	whole grains, liver, avocados, bananas, fish, poultry, meat
(vitamin B_{12})	6.0 unigrams	meat, dairy products, eggs, organ meats (no plant sources)
(folic acid)	400 unigrams	green vegetables, organ meats, wheat, cereals, wheat

	Recommended daily amount	Best sources
		germ, legumes
(vitamin C)	60 milligrams	citrus and berry fruits, green vegetables, tomatoes, potatoes, melons
(vitamin D)	400 I.U.	oily fish, fortified milk, egg yolks
(vitamin E)	30 I.U.	vegetable oils, wheat germ, cereals, bread, liver, eggs, legumes

Figures from the U.S. Recommended Daily Allowances (U.S. R.D.A.) for adults and children over four years of age with the exception of fiber (National Cancer Institute); fat, protein, and carbohydrates (based on National Research Council's Guidelines).

So you can see that many of the foods we often worry about eating are the ones that are best at providing the nutrients we need for good health. And because the nutrients we need are so widely spread among the foods available to us, the crucial factor in good nutrition is to get variety into your diet.

On The Junk Food Diet, that important nutritional balancing act works very well, indeed. Let's

look at the foods and nutrients that have caused—
and continue to cause—the most uproar in recent
years, sort out the realities from the myths, and see
just how The Junk Food Diet copes with the official
recommendations.

FAT

By the late 1970s our fat consumption was over
40 percent of our total energy intake. Thirty percent is the new level to aim for. The other thing we
should try to do is eat less saturated fat (the kind
found in animal and dairy products) and more
mono- and poly-unsaturated fats (the kind found in
plants).

Now, for anyone who wants to lose weight, to cut
down on fat a little is sensible, as fat contains more
calories (9 per gram) than either carbohydrate or
protein (both 4 per gram). But cutting down a little
is what we're talking about here. That 30 percent
goal—or a weight-loss target—in no way means
that we have to give up our favorite meats, cheeses,
milk, and so on.

You could probably achieve the 30 percent figure
by doing nothing more than cutting visible fat off
your meat before you eat it and using a low-fat margarine and mayonnaise in your sandwiches instead
of butter straight from the fridge (when fat is cool
and hard, you can't spread it thin). On The Junk
Food Diet you will cut down your fat intake to well
within acceptable levels because we're reducing the
overall calorie content of your diet and, therefore,
the fat content.

Before we leave the subject of fat, here's a novel
piece of advice that you're not likely to have read

anywhere recently: I don't think it is a particularly good idea to reduce the amount of fat in your diet to much below the official recommendations in the belief that if less is good, virtually none must be even better. In particular, I don't think you should give up red meat. I say that for the following reasons:

Foods that contain animal fat are also excellent sources of some of those vital nutrients we looked at in Table 2. Red meat is second only to liver as the best source of easily absorbed iron. Give up red meat and you'll have to work quite hard, especially if you're female, to get enough iron in your diet—chicken and fish contain little. Red meat is also an important source of vitamin B_{12}, and this is why vegetarians who eat neither meat nor dairy products have to be careful to get enough of this vitamin.

Lean beef, pork, and lamb all contain a high proportion of protein.

Contrary to what people think, the fat in red meat isn't all the saturated kind. Far from it. Mono- and poly-unsaturated fat account for more than two-thirds of the fat in meat. And if you choose your red meat wisely, you are not getting a very high-fat food, in any case. Neither does it appear advisable to try to raise the amount of poly-unsaturated fat (such as corn, safflower, or soybean oil) that you eat either. Major trials have shown that while these fats lower blood-cholesterol levels, thus reducing the risk of CHD, they probably increase the risk from other diseases. Much more research needs to be done, but meanwhile—take it easy!

SUGAR

Long before fat became public enemy number one, sugar was the nutritional bad guy. There were two main reasons.

First, it is the only food that contains no nutrients apart from energy. Nothing but calories! And at 112 calories per ounce, it is quite high in those calories, too.

Second, the evidence incriminating sugar as a major cause of tooth decay is strong.

You may also have heard that sugar is physically addictive, a kind of drug. It is true that sweet foods are the ones most likely to tempt you to eat when you aren't hungry (how many desserts have you succumbed to after claiming you were full?). It is also true that if you eat a high-sugar sweet or snack when you are hungry rather than a more balanced meal or snack, the sugar sets off a chain reaction in your body that has the end result of lowering your blood-sugar level—and helping you to feel you need more sugar. However, this doesn't add up to addiction, and despite the near catalog of complaints against sugar, I still believe that you can enjoy a certain amount of sweet food—even if you're dieting —without feeling guilty.

The Junk Food Diet's message is that sugar is no big deal—if you want some, you can have it, but in a sensible way. I've made sure you get all the nutrients you need for good health within a certain calorie level, and then I've put a fairly generous calorie allowance on top for whatever sugary items you fancy. I also give guidelines on how and when to eat sweet foods, for the sake of your teeth as well as your health. (If you don't have a sweet tooth, use those calories for other treats instead.)

SALT

Although it is quite true that most of us eat a lot more salt than the 1/10 of a teaspoon per day our bodies actually need (in average circumstances) for good health, it is not true to say that salt is a direct cause of high blood pressure or that a drastic reduction in its consumption would result in any particular health benefits for the majority of us. All that has been proved is that if you do suffer from high blood pressure (hypertension) and you cut down your salt intake, your blood pressure may be lowered.

It is estimated that one in five Americans will be at risk for hypertension, and lowering salt intake would be a good idea for those people. (A visit to your doctor to clarify your degree of risk by having a blood-pressure reading will help you and your doctor decide whether you are one of those who would benefit from a low-salt diet.) For the remaining 80 percent of us, it should be more than adequate to cut our consumption to 6 grams or so a day, as the National Research Council Diet and Health Report recommended. If, as most of us probably do, you have been eating around 12 grams a day, that represents a 50 percent cut, which, in fact, is not difficult to achieve. Let's look at the sources of the salt in our daily diets. One-third occurs naturally in our food: for example, in meat, fish, in vegetables, and even in fruit. One-third is added during food processing not only to foods that taste salty, such as smoked bacon and corned beef, but also to a wide variety of other foods, such as breakfast cereals, canned soups, canned vegetables, pickles, tomato ketchup, and bread. One-third is the salt we add ourselves, in cooking and at the table.

On The Junk Food Diet it is easy to cut your salt intake, if you want to, simply by not adding salt to your meals at the table, and by gradually reducing the amount you add while you are cooking. It is easy to cut down even more, if you like, by choosing lower-salt or no-salt items in the supermarket. And more about that in Chapter 4.

If you don't like the idea of cutting down a little on your salt, all I can tell you is that I did exactly that after twenty-five years of eating a lot of salt— and within only two days I found the small reductions I was making completely acceptable. See the High-Salt Foods Table, Table 9, pp. 238.

FIBER

The fiber mania reached such a level of lunacy several years ago that I began to wonder whether the food manufacturers were going to start adding bran to cheese, ice cream, and sherbet in a bid to increase sales. Fiber was the nutritional star of the decade.

Now that the excitement has died down a little, the population falls into two camps—those who stick with whole-grain cereals and dried beans and swear by fiber as a cure for almost everything; and those who adore white spaghetti and white rice and would do almost anything to avoid eating a prune.

If you fall into the latter category, are you doing yourself untold harm? Probably not.

It is a fact that if you suffer from constipation and then increase the amount of fiber-rich foods in your diet, the constipation will almost always be cured. A fiber-rich diet is also useful in preventing or minimizing associated problems such as irritable bowel, diverticulitis (when swellings develop in the walls of the large intestine—a disease common in people over fifty), and hemorrhoids, said to affect up to 10 percent of the population. But all the other cases for fiber, especially as a prevention against heart disease, are still the subject of debate. If you are in normal health without the above problems, it could be that you are already getting plenty of fiber in your diet—and increasing it won't achieve anything.

Few of us actually need more than the recommended 30 grams a day: and very high intakes of bran may impede your body's ability to absorb calcium, iron, and zinc, all three of which are essential minerals. So again, don't think that if some is good, more must be better.

In any case, you don't have to eat lentils and brown rice every day in order to get adequate amounts of fiber. Although it doesn't occur in animal products, only in plants, there is fiber in all kinds of food—yes, even in white spaghetti and white rice! You can eat plenty of "junk" food and still get all the fiber you need, fiber that will help you to lose weight because it will help you to feel full and satisfied. Look down the list in Table 3 and you're bound to find some foods that you like. On The Junk Food Diet, you pick and choose your fiber foods to suit yourself. The set diets contain on average 25 grams of fiber per day, with extra optional.

Table 3

FIBER CONTENT OF SELECTED FOODS

peas, black-eyed, cooked, 1 cup	24.80 grams
beans, baked, 1/2 cup	10.97 grams
peas, green, cooked, 1 cup	10.74 grams
beans, lima, cooked, 1 cup	8.70 grams
beans, black, cooked, 1 cup	7.20 grams
brussels sprouts, cooked, 1 cup	7.20 grams
chili with beans, 1 cup	5.10 grams
potato, baked, with skin, 1	4.92 grams
beans, green, cooked, 1 cup	4.57 grams
onions, cooked, 1 cup	4.40 grams
spinach, cooked, 1 cup	4.00 grams
vegetables, mixed, canned, 1 cup	3.91 grams
corn, cooked, 1 ear	3.62 grams
carrots, raw, grated, 1 cup	3.58 grams
onions, raw, sliced, 1 cup	3.52 grams
potato, mashed, 1 cup	3.40 grams
strawberries, 1 cup	3.20 grams
cantaloupe, raw, 1/2	2.67 grams
potato chips, 10	2.40 grams
lettuce, 1/6 crisp head	2.03 grams

mushrooms, raw, 1 cup	1.80 grams
spaghetti, 1 cup, plain	1.49 grams
peanut butter, 1 tablespoon	1.10 grams
corn tortilla, 1	1.00 grams
celery, stalk, raw	.87 grams

CALCIUM

Calcium is another nutrient to come under the spotlight. Its role in minimizing or preventing osteoporosis, a debilitating weakening of the bones that primarily affects one in four women past menopause, has been the subject of much media attention, but once again, there is no absolute agreement among the experts about exactly how big a role calcium plays, nor about exactly how much calcium we should be getting in our diets.

The Recommended Dietary Allowance is *800 milligrams* for women. Some sources say we should strive for 1,200 to 1,500 milligrams per day.

One fact is certain: An adequate calcium intake is essential to make, and keep, strong bones. The denser your bones, the less trouble osteoporosis should cause in old age. And on The Junk Food Diet, your richest source of calcium—dairy foods—isn't limited drastically. Besides dairy products, you can get calcium in lots of different foods—everything from sardines to taco chips. A quick look at Table 4 will yield some surprising sources.

Table 4

CALCIUM CONTENT OF FAVORITE FOODS

potato chips, 10	5 milligrams
potatoes, french fries, 10	10
tortilla, corn, 1	42
pita bread, 1	49
egg, scrambled, 1	54
halibut, cooked, 4 ounces	57
snow pea pods, cooked, 1 cup	67
sweet potatoes, canned, mashed, 1 cup	77
crab leg, 1	80
bread stuffing, from mix, 1 cup	88
diet hot chocolate, 1 serving	89
trout, cooked, 4 ounces	96
English muffin, 1	96
shrimp, canned, 3 ounces	98
scallops, cooked, 3 1/2 ounces	115
cottage cheese, 1 cup	155
Chinese cabbage, cooked, 1 cup	158
oatmeal, cooked, instant, 1 package	163

salmon, canned, with bones, 3 ounces	167 mg
American cheese, 1 slice	200
potatoes, au gratin, from mix, 1 cup	203
Cheddar cheese, 1 ounce	204
broccoli, cooked, 1 spear	205
spinach, cooked, 1 cup	245
Swiss cheese, 1 ounce	272
sardines, canned, with bones, 3 ounces	371

Table 5

VITAMIN C CONTENT OF FAMILIAR FOODS

potatoes, french fries, 10	5 mg
potato chips, 10	8
lettuce, 1 cup	10
apple, 1 large	12
orange soda, diet	18
pineapple, raw, diced, 1 cup	24
tangerine, 1	26
blackberries, 1 cup	30

sherbet, 2% fat	31 mg
grapefruit, 1/2 medium	41
asparagus spears, 1 cup	44
cauliflower, cooked, 1 cup	69
orange, 1	70
grapefruit juice, 1 cup	72
kiwi, 1	74
pea pods, cooked, 1 cup	77
strawberries, 1 cup	84
orange juice, 1 cup	86
papaya, raw, 1 cup	92
cantaloupe, 1/2 medium	113
broccoli, cooked, 1 spear	113
Hi-C punch, 12 ounces	120
pepper, 1, sweet, red, raw	141

VITAMINS

On a varied diet, even a low-calorie one, you're unlikely to go short of vitamins. Every food you eat, apart from white sugar, contains something that's good for you!

A regular supply is vital, as your body doesn't store it, and apart from a little in liver and milk, vitamin C is found only in fruit and vegetables.

Junk-food lovers often have an aversion to fruits and vegetables. But if you're a greens-hater, you can still get plenty of vitamin C: How about green peppers or potatoes? Even fries are a good source, and so are tomatoes.

If you're not keen on any vegetables at all, try fruit: Soft fruits, melons, and all citrus fruits are great sources of vitamin C. You don't like fruit either? How about fruit juice? One half cup of orange juice gives you all the vitamin C you need each day.

And don't forget, your fruit and vegetables don't have to be fresh: frozen and canned both contain vitamin C, too. On The Junk Food Diet I'll make sure you get your vitamin C one way or another!

FOOD PROCESSING

Processed food was frequently mentioned in my survey (see Chapter 1) as a prime example of what was meant by "junk food." And yet processed foods make up one-half to three-quarters of the American diet! If this figure sounds high, it's simply because a large proportion of food in its "natural" state isn't fit to eat. Processing, for instance, turns cereal grains into bread and breakfast cereals. It also makes available to us a gigantic variety of foods that would otherwise be unavailable—out-of-season vegetables can be frozen and out-of-season fruits can be canned, for instance.

It is true that there are some highly processed products on sale that are low in nutrients and high on that other scapegoat of the 1980s—additives. Long-shelf-life cakes, pies, and pastries are probably as near to genuine junk as you will find—and yet, even so, a slice of "eat within two years" fake-cream-filled sponge cake or a pack or two of instant-pudding mix now and then is not going to harm you.

Food-additive intolerance appears to be yet another area for doubt. A recent large study involving 10 percent of the entire population of a large British town resulted in only three people showing "clinically definable" intolerance.

Despite trial results such as these, food additives are a very sensitive area, and this is why the food manufacturers are busy removing more and more additives from their products. In fact, they are doing their best to ensure that the quality of canned and convenience foods is higher than ever before.

You could eat a perfectly healthy diet without ever having to go near a fresh food again. Table 6 gives an example of a day's healthy eating without any fresh foods in it at all. (Chapter 4 deals in more detail with processed foods and your diet; Chapter 11 deals specifically with children and food processing.)

Table 6

A DAY'S HEALTHY EATING,* INCLUDING NO FRESH FOODS

Breakfast
1 cup shredded wheat, served with 1 cup reconstituted dry milk, 1/2 cup orange juice, canned, 1 crispbread with 2 teaspoons honey.

Lunch
3 ounce can tuna in water, drained, 1/2 cup canned three-bean salad, 4-ounce serving vanilla ice cream, 1/4 can peach halves in juice or syrup, drained, 1 can iced tea.

Snack
1 small box raisins

Evening meal
4-ounce hamburger (frozen), broiled and drained,
1/2 cup instant mashed potatoes, 3/4 cup mixed
carrots and peas, canned, individual serving
canned chocolate pudding.

Snack
1-ounce bag potato chips

Throughout day
3/4 cup reconstituted dry milk in tea and coffee

---

*For a 120-pound adult woman on a maintenance diet.

This day's diet provides: 1,700 calories (some
women may need more than this to maintain their
ideal body weight); a low-fat content of just over 30
percent of the total energy intake; 27.3 grams of
fiber, 18 percent of the total energy intake in protein; 48 percent energy intake in carbohydrates; 66
grams of vitamin C; 820 milligrams of calcium; 9
milligrams of iron; 7,258 unigrams of vitamin A;
0.62 milligrams of vitamin B_1; 1.47 milligrams of
vitamin B_2; 20.17 milligrams of vitamin B_3. The total added sodium content of the diet is 2,500 milligrams.

Healthy junk indeed!

TAKEOUT FOOD

Finally, the remaining great subject of debate among students of healthy eating is fast foods—are they of poor nutritional value, and how often should you eat them?

All takeout foods fit into one of three categories:

1. many good points and few, or no, bad ones;
2. some good points and some bad ones;
3. many bad points and few good ones.

No takeout meal on earth can be described as 100 percent junk. But how to sort out the excellent takeout meal from the poor one? I've devised a checklist of good points to look out for, with the corresponding bad points.

Good	*Bad*
very recently prepared/ cooked	been prepared/kept warm a long time
if fried, fresh, clean, unsaturated oil used at correct temperature	fried in animal fat/ overused oil at too low a temperature
contains at least 10 percent protein	contains very little protein
contains reasonable amount of fiber	contains little fiber
contains not more than 30% fat	high in fat
contains vitamin C	no vitamin C
high nutrition-to-calories ratio	low nutrition-to-calories ratio

low to average salt con-   high salt content
    tent

Scoring 1 for every good point and 1 for every bad
one, let's look at a few popular takeout foods.

Hamburger in white bun with ketchup, mustard, and a
pickle from a national burger chain

Scores 5 good points and 2 bad (low in fiber and
contains no vitamin C). Second category doesn't apply. So, on average, a hamburger is a good takeout
food. (If you eat food from a lot of takeouts, it's always wise to get it from a national chain because
food turnover is high and certain standards always
apply: For example, food is prepared and cooked
when your order is placed whenever possible, and
standard ingredients, portion sizes, and cooking
methods are standard.)

Mexican food

Scores 8 good points and no bad ones if you steer
clear of large amounts refried beans and toppings
like guacamole, sour cream, and extra cheese.

Pizza from national chain

Depending upon the variety you choose, pizza scores
from 4 to 8 good points and 0 to 4 bad ones. Some
pizzas contain more fiber and vitamin C than others, and some are quite high in fat and/or salt content, largely depending on the amount and type of
cheese in them.

Fried chicken

Fried chicken varies enormously in its nutritional value from shop to shop. A portion of chicken in batter with fries from a "greasy spoon" with low turnover may give you a very high-calorie, high-saturated-fat, low-vitamin-C meal with hardly any chicken (therefore hardly any protein) inside the batter. Bad-point score could rate up to 6! On the other hand, a standardized, well-cooked portion of chicken in a thin coating of batter, and fries, from a chain could yield all good points and no bad ones.

Chinese food

Chinese takeout shops are the hardest of all to categorize because there is no standardization. But in general you can use common sense to get a reasonably good estimate of good and bad scores. If a beef stir fry is swimming in visible fat, for instance, it is safe to assume it is high in fat altogether.

Is it sensible to indulge in takeout food or not? Yes, I think it is! Takeouts are by no means the nutritional bad guys they are often made out to be. Not by a long shot. But, of course, no one can force you to buy a balanced meal: a hamburger, thick shake, and apple pie, for instance, may well put your day's diet in total disarray, whereas a hamburger, orange juice, and a small order of french fries might have been the perfect meal.

TAKEOUT AND FAST-FOOD TIPS

- Choose a popular busy national chain where you're likely to get the best nutritional value.
- Takeout foods that include no freshly cooked french fries and no fruit or fruit juice, vegetable or salad will contain no vitamin C. Add a piece of fresh fruit yourself, or make sure you get C-rich foods at another time during the day.
- Don't think of a fast food just as a small snack in between main meals; think of it as a meal in itself.
- Use common sense when choosing a complete takeout meal. Get some carbohydrates (bun, rice, bread) plus some protein (meat, fish, cheese, egg), and no more than one high-fat item (pastry, chips, thick shakes)—and you can't go far wrong.

So there you have virtually all the good news about your diet. But here's some news that may cheer you up even more, as you are about to embark on your diet to shed that unwanted weight.

If you lose weight you'll be doing your health the biggest favor of all.

In the fight against chronic illness and complaints of many kinds—including heart disease—a slim body is your greatest ally. Being overweight can cause or aggravate all the following conditions; being thin will help you to avoid them, minimize them—or even cure some of them:

- heart disease, strokes, and high blood pressure
- mid-life-onset diabetes.
- arthritis and other joint disorders

In addition, increasing degrees of obesity in men are statistically linked with increased risk of colon, rectal, and prostate cancers. Increasing degrees of obesity in women are statistically linked with increased risk of breast, uterine, and cervical cancer.

The fact is that it is being overweight, and not specific dietary components, that is the biggest threat to our twentieth-century Western health. In other words, it's not so much what you eat as *how much.*

Do yourself a favor and lose that weight.

A SUMMARY OF WHAT YOU'VE READ IN CHAPTER 2

- Healthy eating does not mean you have to give up fat, sugar, salt, and all your favorite foods.
- Healthy eating is as much about getting enough of all the nutrients you need as it is about cutting down on others.
- Fat-containing foods can be a useful part of your diet.
- You can enjoy a certain amount of sugar in your diet without feeling guilty.
- Salt may not be a health hazard for most people, but it's easy to cut down on the salt in your diet if you are an "at risk" person.
- You can live quite healthfully on a diet of processed foods.
- By no means are all takeout foods poor foods.
- One of the best ways to help your health is to lose weight.

✤ 3. ✤

Eating to Lose—
Myth and Reality

IF YOU HAD LOST AN OUNCE FOR EVERY LUDICROUS dieting "fact" that I have read, been told, or overheard during the past decade, you wouldn't need to lose weight now, that's for certain.

So much nonsense is talked about and written about the subject of dieting that it is amazing that people can keep finding new things to make up. Yet find them they do. And that is why I want to take some time here to "clear the decks" and clear your head of all those half-remembered "truths" and half-forgotten myths so that you won't be sidetracked or ambushed when you begin dieting this time.

Let's look at how you are most likely to have come by ridiculous dieting advice.

DIETING FOLKLORE

One of the earliest "dieting facts" was first announced around twenty years ago when, so we were told, a grapefruit eaten before every meal would help you lose weight because it "burned up" the calories in your food. Remember?

Well, surprise, surprise; just when we all thought the grapefruit theory had been consigned to the dieting trash can, it had a revival, this time in the form of grapefruit pills, marketed most successfully a couple of years ago—presumably because all of us old enough to have been around the first time had forgotten that they didn't work.

I think dieting myths are a bit like a favorite pair of worn-out slippers: We know they're useless but we don't want to throw them out. Foods that are supposed to "burn up" other foods or the fat in your own body are at the top of the list. I know people who swear that protein, eaten in the form of a steak or a chicken leg, for example, "burns off" your fat, and that is why a high-protein diet slims you down. But only if you eat the protein with no carbohydrates, folks! (So what happens if you eat protein plus grapefruit—a carbohydrate—I wonder?) Talking of high-protein diets, I also often hear that these work because the body can't convert excess protein into fat. (It can, and it does, if you aren't getting enough calories from the carbohydrate foods.)

You've probably got some more folklore of your own. Well, now you know what to do with it.

SCIENTIFIC THEORIES

"Nutritional breakthrough!" "Amazing new diet theory!" "Scientifically tested way to lose!"

I have hundreds of diet books on my office shelves that promise dieters the earth and quote pseudo-scientific tests and theories. Over the past decade or more, various authors have told us, as if it were a proven fact rather than a mere theory, that, for example, our bodies burn up calories better if we eat nothing except fruit until lunchtime. We have been told that the only way to get thin is to eat what we like, but in a certain order, so that the different types of food don't mix. We've been urged to take supplements of amino acids to alter our metabolic rates. And we've been assured that by taking large doses of certain vitamins we will also raise our metabolic rates.

Now I tell you that all these theories are, at best, unproven, and, at worst, absolute rubbish. You may well lose weight by following a diet that heralds itself with pages of scientific-sounding mumbo-jumbo. But you will lose weight because the diet is low in calories, not because its author has made the one amazing breakthrough your digestive system has been waiting for all these years!

The famous Beverly Hills Diet, for instance, sold us the crazy idea of "combining" foods in a certain order and eating masses of "enzyme-producing" pineapples and the like. But the diet actually worked to get the pounds falling off you fast because it was very, very low in calories.

So don't be fooled by an important-sounding diet that will have you scurrying around looking for out-of-season fruits or expensive pill supplements. You don't need them.

"BUT YOU MUST . . ."

The sort of advice you are likely to get from friends—who are probably only trying to be helpful and encouraging—most frequently takes the form of things you "must" and "mustn't" eat when you're dieting.

They will be horrified if they see you tucking into

a bag of chips or enjoying a glass of wine. They will creep guiltily off to the vending machine and hide conspicuously behind the filing cabinet when they want to eat a candy bar, never dreaming that you can actually eat one yourself if you want to.

The fact is that there are no hard and fast rules about what you must and mustn't eat on a weight-loss diet—only, I repeat, that you should take in fewer calories over the course of a day, or a week, than your body needs to maintain its current weight.

It's worth taking a closer look at the most-often uttered "musts" and "mustn'ts"; the kind of prejudices you'll be up against from everyone—including the family doctor, if you should ever happen to ask for advice on weight loss from that quarter. Not one of them stands up to close examination.

Read on—carefully—so you'll know exactly what to say in answer to the people who will be trying (in a well-meaning way, of course!) to make your life miserable while you diet.

"You must eat lots of salad when you're dieting."

Just why salad has gotten its reputation as obligatory food for people wishing to lose weight, I'm not sure. True, lettuce, cucumber, tomatoes, celery, and so on are very low in calories, but apart from that distinction, your traditional salad has little to recommend it. It will provide some vitamin C and some fiber, but it is by no means the best source of either, or of any other nutrient. It doesn't fill you up and it is so boring that many dieters, driven to distraction by their compulsory salad with their steak or their ham or their cheese, fall into what I call the Mayonnaise Syndrome. They dollop on great spoonfuls of dressing—be it mayonnaise, Thousand Island, French dressing, or blue-cheese dressing. Ah! That tastes better! But whichever dressing you choose, you can be sure of one thing—you just turned your goodie-goodie salad of around 25 calories into a 150-calories-plus plateful. The irony is that you could have had all the mashed potatoes you wanted, say, or two slices of bread instead.

If you don't like salad—don't feel obliged to eat it! Nothing dreadful will happen to you if you don't, I promise!

"You must eat more fish and poultry."

Steamed or grilled white fish is probably second only to lettuce in sending any would-be dieter off on a chocolate binge. If you're not a fish lover, apply the same philosophy. If you force yourself to eat it, you'll only end up breaking your diet. And if you do eat it, you're likely to pile on the tartar sauce or make up for your deprivation with a larger-than-average helping of french fries.

Yes, fish is a good source of protein, and even if you can't face more than the occasional cod or sole fillet, you may find you like trout or rich and meaty swordfish, for instance. But by no means is all fish as low in calories as cod, sole, and haddock are, at around 22 calories per ounce each. Salmon and sardines are around 50 per ounce, sardines 60, and so is mackerel. So don't be fooled into thinking that all fish is lower in calories than meat. It isn't.

Very lean beef (a lean cut, reasonably well roasted or grilled and trimmed of visible fat) is only 40 calories per ounce. Lean ground beef, cooked, then drained of fat, is the same. So, you see, there's nothing to say you shouldn't eat red meat on your diet. And with butchers paying more and more attention to giving us less fat meat all the time, you shouldn't feel guilty about eating a burger or a steak instead of a piece of fish or chicken. Chicken meat, by the way, is about 50 calories per ounce, without its skin. With its skin, it goes up to 60— proving nothing except that you should eat chicken only because you like it and not because someone told you it's less fattening than red meat!

"You must eat a good breakfast when you're dieting."

If you happen to be one of the many who doesn't eat breakfast and then you are told by some bullyboy of a diet that you must, first you will feel resentful, and second, you will, more than likely, put on weight.

Some people (and I am one of them) are genuinely not hungry when they first get up. It seems silly, then, if you are trying to cut back on the amount you eat, to stuff several hundred calories down yourself at a time when you could gladly do without them. Much better to save the calories for a snack later in the day when you do feel hungry.

So why do so many people, nutritionists and weight-loss club leaders included, say you should eat a "good breakfast"? If you're dieting, the theory is that if you miss breakfast, you will undoubtedly feel starved by mid-morning and binge then.

It is also claimed that you will feel faint and lack concentration throughout the morning if you don't eat breakfast. Well, I feel all right, but only you know how you feel, and whether or not eating something before 9 A.M. helps you feel any better. Probably, if you always eat breakfast and feel hungry at that time of day, then you would suffer if you gave it up. If you're a non-breakfast eater, then for heaven's sake, don't start now!

"You must re-educate your palate to diet successfully."

In certain cases "re-educating" your palate can be helpful. For example, it takes only a fair degree of willpower over a three-week period to change from being a confirmed user of two spoonfuls of sugar in your coffee to someone who makes a face if she detects as much as a few grains of sugar in the cup. Similarly, when you reduce the amount of salt you use in cooking and at the table, it is amazing how quickly your previous "normal" amount tastes quite awful. So, helping your taste buds to get used to less-sweet tastes, for instance, can be very useful.

But no amount of "palate conditioning" will work to help you lose unless you re-educate your mind first! You've got to want to lose weight, and you've got to be convinced that you can do it—more about that in Chapter 5.

"You mustn't eat fried foods when on a diet."

There's no *mustn't* and no *must* about it, but you can if you want to.

Although on The Junk Food Diet you will be reducing the overall fat content of what you eat, that isn't to say you can't eat some fat, and some of the fat can be in the form of fried foods, if that is what you really like.

Some fried foods aren't as fattening as people will have you believe. Take fried eggs. One average raw egg contains about 80 calories. Fried in hot oil and well drained on a slotted spoon before being served, it will contain only about 120 calories. That's 40 calories' worth of fat, or around 4.5 grams—less than a teaspoonful of oil.

By cooking foods quickly in very hot oil you can save a lot of calories. Put frozen fries into oil that isn't hot enough and they'll sit around soaking up the fat until they start cooking. They will be twice as high in calories as thick-cut fries cooked for a little time in really hot fat. And frying big items rather than small ones can save you hundreds of calories—forget fried scallops and go for a big chunk of cod!

Shallow frying certain foods can actually be no more fattening then broiling them. For instance, if you start bacon off in a warm, non-stick pan and gradually heat it up until its own fat starts to run out, then turn the heat up and fry it until the bacon is golden and crisp, then drain the bacon well when you serve it, it will have no more calories than if you had broiled it. This also applies to sausages (well cooked), steak, and burgers. When fatty meat cooks, by whatever means, it loses fat; it doesn't absorb it.

Last, stir-frying is a great way to fry if you're watching your calorie intake. You don't have to have a wok; a non-stick pan will do. Add a couple of teaspoons of oil, your favorite thinly sliced meat and vegetables, and, if you keep stirring while you cook over a high heat, add perhaps a little stock or soy sauce along the way, you have a dish that smells, looks, and tastes wickedly high in calories but isn't at all.

"You mustn't snack between meals."

Not true. Not only is snacking between meals not harmful to your diet; it could be an advantage!

First, to know that you can have something to eat other than at breakfast, lunch, and dinner is very comforting when you're dieting. It stops you from feeling deprived. If you aren't "allowed" to snack, you are much more likely to cheat and eat that candy bar anyway.

The anti-snackers say that between-meal snacks will make you fat because you eat them as extras, in addition to your ordinary meals. But of course that doesn't have to be the case at all. The Junk Food Diet will show you how to include snacks within your day's allowances!

Second, several small meals a day will help to keep your metabolism working at top efficiency; in other words, you may get thin a little more quickly by eating, say, five snacks rather than two big meals a day.

So if you enjoy snack eating, don't try to change!

"You mustn't eat starchy foods when you're dieting."

I can hardly believe it when I hear it, but I still get dieters telling me proudly that they are on a high-protein diet and being "good" by cutting out bread and potatoes.

So if someone is plugging that idea to you as the best way to diet, ignore him or her. The "starch" foods—like rice, pasta, bread, and potatoes—are a valuable part, both practically and nutritionally, of your weight-loss diet.

Potatoes cooked plainly have only 25 calories or less per ounce, compared with 120 for a "protein" food like Cheddar cheese. Cooked rice and pasta have 35 calories per ounce, and bread has 60 to 70. So it's the starchy foods that help fill you up when you are on a diet, as well as providing vital nutrients, without giving you too many calories. They are the backbone of any decent diet that isn't going to leave you ravenously hungry, and, as you will find out, on The Junk Food Diet I don't believe in your being ravenous at all.

"You mustn't drink alcohol while on a diet."

There are certain people who shouldn't drink alcohol whether or not they are dieting. For example, if you are under medical orders not to do so, if you are taking certain prescription medications, if you are pregnant or if you are trying to conceive, do not drink alcohol.

Otherwise, if a glass of wine with your evening meal, a can of beer after work, or a Scotch when you get home is your idea of a treat, then I see no reason at all why you shouldn't continue to enjoy it while on a diet.

Alcoholic drinks aren't that high in calories: a glass of wine is about 90 calories, a single shot (jigger) of liquor is 50, and a 12-ounce can or bottle of light beer is about 100 calories.

On The Junk Food Diet, your "daily treats" allowance can be taken in alcohol, if you like, without your feeling guilty, because I have made sure that the limit is within guidelines for good health. I will also show you how to cope with those special occasions, like your birthday, when one glass or two just doesn't seem enough!

Of course, if you have been a habitual 6-pack-a-night man, then that could explain why you need to lose some weight, and you are going to have to make some compromises here.

Certainly, if you've been used to having more than a couple of drinks a day on a regular basis, then I would suggest cutting down, not only to help you lose weight, but also for the sake of your general health. I managed to more than halve my own consumption of my favorite drink, white wine, by mixing it, at first half and half, and then a third to two-thirds, with sparkling mineral water. I now find I actually prefer the watered-down version!

Here are some more tips to help you control the amount you drink:

- Drink your fill of water before you start on alcohol so that you're not thirsty.
- Sip, don't gulp.
- Put your glass down between sips.
- Try alcohol-free wine or beer.

Heavy drinking comes down to being a habit in most cases, just as overeating does, so if you can find easy ways to break the habit, the rest is simple.

If none of my tips works, or if you can't even bring yourself to try any of them, consider getting professional help.

"You shouldn't eat cakes, cookies and ice cream on a diet."

It is true that you could blow a whole day's calorie allowance on a couple of items if you chose unwisely. For instance, 1,000 calories would be gone in a flash if you decided to eat one good slice of cheesecake and a big helping of Black Forest cake with ice cream.

On the other hand, you could have a slice of sponge cake, a couple of sugar cookies, and a frozen yogurt and still have enough calories left over to have a nutritious day's eating on 1,000 calories a day.

A little of what you crave does do you good, so don't try to diet by cutting out all the things you like best. It just won't work.

"You shouldn't touch chocolate—one taste will send you on a binge."

Not if you are on The Junk Food Diet, it won't!

I know that many people think of chocolate as a demon to be banished from their lives before it overtakes them completely, but it can be bullied into shape and take its place legitimately in your diet.

The secret is to allow for it within your weight-loss program, enjoy it, savor it, eat it—and don't feel guilty. Then get on with your life and your diet.

What does end in a binge—be it a binge of chocolate or sweets, bread or oatmeal cookies—is a long spell of deprivation.

You know the scene. You start a diet, one of the many that limits your choice of food, especially of the one food you really like. You stick to the diet for a few days, even a week or two. You're proud of your strong willpower and your few pounds of weight loss. You've said no to your favorite food—you've won the battle!

Then, halfway through day three, or day seven, or day ten, for no reason that you can really explain, you surrender. You walk into the kitchen quite intent upon grabbing a piece of Melba toast and an apple, and somehow you walk out with a handful of chocolate-covered cookies. Or you pop into the corner shop for a magazine on your way home from work, and without even knowing you did it, you buy two Mars Bars (maybe three). They are all gone by the time you get home. And then, feeling like a failure, you will sit down and polish off a plate of brownies.

You won a battle but you lost the war. "What does it matter anymore?" you say. "That's one more diet down the drain. I just can't diet. I haven't got the willpower." And it's a long, long time before you think about losing weight again.

Yet it's not your willpower that's at fault, it's the diet—for making you exercise superhuman willpower in the first place. The deprivation method of dieting can't work for most of us for more than a few days.

For more about how you can eat chocolate—and all the other "binge" foods—while you diet, and for more about how you can stop thinking of a weight-loss diet as a battleground where temptation will always beat you, turn to Chapter 5.

A SUMMARY OF WHAT YOU'VE READ
IN CHAPTER 3

- Think very carefully before accepting advice you read or hear about dieting; it's probably wrong!
- There are no hard and fast rules about what you should or shouldn't eat on a diet; as long as you reduce your overall food consumption, you will lose weight.
- It is not true that you must eat salad, lots of fish and poultry, a good breakfast, regular meals, or a great deal of high-fiber food in order to lose weight.
- It is not true that you shouldn't eat fried foods, starchy foods, in-between-meal snacks, cakes, ice cream, or cookies.
- The only successful way to lose weight is to include your favorite foods in the diet.

❖ 4. ❖

Supermarkets— User-Friendly Shopping

HAVE YOU EVER WONDERED WHY THE PEOPLE YOU SEE going in and out of health-food stores don't appear to be any healthier than the rest of us?

There is certainly no proof that people who avoid supermarkets live longer and healthier lives than the 75 percent of us who happily push that giant cart once a week.

And I'm not surprised. I believe that supermarket shopping is by far the best bet for anyone who wants his or her diet to be nutritious, low-calorie, and tasty. And here are my reasons why:

- Virtually everything that can be bought at a health-food store (with the possible exception of a handful of specialty vegetarian items) can be bought at the supermarket chains, but the opposite is far from true, even when it comes to "healthy" items. For instance, where a health-food store may offer one or, at most, two varieties of whole-grain cereal, the supermarket will offer five or more. There is far more choice of everything.

- The supermarkets have a high turnover of produce so you can be sure of finding fresh foods. Quality is also closely monitored and standards are high.

- Fresh fruits and vegetables are kept in perfect condition in supermarkets. Having been packed and transported correctly, they are then displayed for sale in cool conditions, often with specially dimmed lighting, which helps preserve maximum vitamin content. Most health-food stores don't have the facilities or the room to do this, and produce kept in warm, light (sunlight is worst of all) conditions, and perhaps kept for a week or more when business is slow, will lose a large amount of vitamin C—a vitamin vital to your good health. A good-quality supermarket tomato is worth twenty organically grown but badly stored health-food store tomatoes.

- Supermarkets have a wide range of food suitable for dieters, almost all of which are labeled with calorie information. Portions are standardized and controlled, and everything from low-calorie alternatives to high-calorie foods are always stocked.

- Most supermarkets even provide calorie information on the "naughty" foods like pre-packed cakes and pastry products, so you can easily build them into your diet. And if you want even more information—on fat or sugar content, for instance—that's provided for many foods, too.

- Most supermarkets have additional nutritional information available for you: full calorie-counted lists of products, diet booklets, family meal planners, healthy-eating leaflets, recipe leaflets, and so on.

In addition to all those plus-points, prices on comparable items are almost always lower at supermarkets, with the possible exception of some items sold "loose," such as shelled nuts, herbs, and spices. So stop feeling guilty every time you pass by the health-food store. Instead, I'm going to take you now on a special dieters' guided tour of the much-maligned supermarkets to show you exactly how much they can help you on your diet. But first, to avoid or get around the few pitfalls you will come across as you shop, take note of these tips:

- **Take a list.** Casual, unplanned, haphazard shopping (whether it's for food or clothes) always results in your getting home with things you didn't want, things you already have more than enough of, and things you wish you could take straight back. If it's clothes, you probably will take them back; if it's food, you'll probably eat it.
- **Don't ever shop when you're hungry.** It is amazing how much more you think you need when you wheel your cart around the aisles just before lunchtime, faint from starvation. Don't do it. Eat your meal. Then do your shopping. You'll save money as well as pounds.
- **If you haven't many items on your list, use a basket, not a cart.**
- **Get tough about special offers.** Even armed with your list, it is tempting to buy two or three packages of cookies just because they are a few cents cheaper this week—even if you don't like that particular kind of cookie! Buy only those items you like or need, things you have room for in the cupboard/fridge/freezer, and things that

won't spoil or rot before you have time to eat
them.

Now let's get on with that tour.

VISITING THE SUPERMARKET

The dairy case

Dieters can certainly forget the long-gone days
when the only choice was natural cottage cheese or
nothing. The manufacturers have done wonders in
producing all kinds of lower-calorie cheeses, and the
best news of all are the reduced-fat versions of our
favorite, such as Cheddar, Swiss, Monterey Jack,
and cheese spreads. Calorie savings range from 25
percent to 50 percent, which will always be explained on the pack. In addition to keeping an eye
out for the supermarket's own brands, look out for
Light n' Lively, Lite Line, and Weight Watchers reduced-calorie cheeses.

Full-fat cream cheese has 100 calories per ounce.
The reduced-fat soft cheeses are very nice—and contain only 80 calories per ounce. Even the dreaded
cottage cheese can be quite nice these days—it
comes in dozens of varieties, and some brands are
very creamy.

More and more of us are turning to skim milk
and away from whole milk. But if you are one of
those people who still finds the taste of skim milk
too thin, it is worth trying low-fat or 1% milk. You
still save 50 calories a cup, and, if no one tells you, I
swear you'll never know the difference! If you use

dried milk powder, don't forget that some have added fat. Read the label carefully.

Moving on to the fats section, you'll see that butter takes up much less space than it did a decade ago, and in its place are all kinds of "spreadables." Some of these, but by no means all of them, contain only half the calories of butter. All these will be clearly labeled "low-fat spread." Some brand names to look for are Mazola, Parkay Diet Soft, Fleischmann's Diet, Weight Watchers. Imitation margarines spread so easily and so thinly that you save even more calories that way, too—butter straight from the fridge doesn't spread, it goes on in chunks.

If you're wondering whether to buy oil instead of butter for cooking, to save calories, oil (all kinds) actually has more calories than butter. At 125 calories per tablespoon it's the highest-calorie food in the world! Corn or sunflower oil is best if you're looking for poly-unsaturates. Olive oil is high in mono-unsaturates and has a lot more flavor than corn, sunflower, or safflower oil. Blended oils often are high in saturated fats—those are the ones to avoid.

The meat counter

If you're dieting there is no need to pass by the red-meat counter. Beef, pork, bacon, and lamb can all be lower in calories than chicken or turkey! This is for two reasons. First, the meat producers are bowing to popular request and producing cows, pigs, and sheep with a higher lean-to-fat ratio. In other words, there is less fat in traditional cuts of meat than there was a decade or so ago. Second, many butchers now prepare the various cuts of meat trimmed of almost all visible fat. Of course, many butchers still stick to their old methods, but the leading supermarkets are one step ahead in the race to give us leaner meat. While they still offer fattier cuts, you will always find a selection of leaner cuts, too. These will be marked either "less than 10 percent fat" or "lean" or "choice," and you should find ground beef, stewing meat, braising meat, fillets, steaks, and cutlets from which to choose.

If you don't find any meat marked "low in fat," simply have a good look at the cuts available and pick one that seems to have the least visible amount of fat. Everyone thinks pork and lamb are fatty, but their lean meat can be no more fattening than chicken at 50 calories an ounce. So the message when buying meat is to avoid the fatty cuts. Belly cuts and breast and shoulder of lamb are among the fattiest there are! Duck, by the way, isn't too bad if it's well cooked. Most of that fat will have melted away into the roasting pan.

The frozen-food case

These are full of good things for dieters. There are dozens of ready meals, all calorie-counted, and most are quite low in calories, too. There's so much variety, with recipes from all over the world, that dieting really becomes fun. They are ideal for cheaters —in order to get second helpings you have to buy two packages.

Other frozen foods ideal for dieters are individual pizzas, French-bread pizzas, individual pies, stir fries, and the various crispy-coated fish, as well as poultry fillets and burgers, all of which can be baked, microwaved, or broiled rather than deep-fried.

Sweet-toothers can choose ice cream as a reasonable low-calorie dessert, but beware the family-sized frozen cakes and tortes unless you really do have a hungry family. Once they're defrosted, you can't cut off just one small slice, can you?

Frozen fruits and vegetables are perfect dieter's fare. If you live alone, you can pour just what you need, so there's no temptation to "finish up the can." And the vitamin C content of frozen fruits and vegetables is high. If you are fed up with fries, you can try the dozens of other potato products, which can be grilled, oven-baked, or microwaved.

Canned foods

Even if you have a freezer, you may want to stock up on some canned meats, fish, fruits, and vegetables—in fact, anything you can get fresh, you can get in a can. If you are one of those people who equates cans with "nasty additives," it's worth thinking again. Canning is a method of preservation in itself, so the addition of further preservatives and anti-oxidants is unnecessary. The quality of canned food depends largely on the quality of the food when it was fresh. And canning doesn't destroy all the vitamin C in fruits and vegetables.

Depending on the product, the can may contain added sugar or salt. But if you look along the shelves you will find low-sugar fruits that will save you some calories. And if you're watching your salt intake, you'll find low-salt alternatives, too.

Jars

Down in the preserves aisle you can find low-calorie
versions of almost all your favorites. There's low-
sugar jam and reduced-oil mayonnaise, both of
them saving 50 percent of the calories. There's oil-
free salad dressing for almost no calories a spoonful,
as opposed to 120.

Dry goods

Don't forget a package of instant mashed potatoes,
some dried fruits and nuts for nibbles, some rice
and pasta for quick meals, and plenty of cereals for
breakfast. You can also find low-calorie sweeteners
to use instead of sugar on your cornflakes or for
your morning coffee. Artificial sweeteners have
come a long way since straight saccharine; the new
generation is hard to distinguish from sugar. That's
why all those calorie-free soft drinks are so good
now—speaking of such, you could put some of those
in your cart, too.

THE ADDITIVES QUESTION

Should you feel that you are doing your body untold harm if you buy packages, jars, or cans of food
with preservatives in them?

A major recent controlled British trial sponsored
by the Ministry of Agriculture has shown that allergic reaction to additives—indeed, to any foods, including natural ones such as wheat—is much rarer
than we have been led to believe. If you know that
you are allergic to a certain food additive, then of
course you should avoid that food or additive. But

999 people out of 1,000 can eat foods containing preservatives and can both feel and be perfectly well and healthy, according to this British study. All additives in food for sale for humans in this country have been approved by the government after extensive tests, and so the blanket idea that all additives are in some way harmful for all people is one you can safely leave behind. Some additives, such as vitamin C and beta-carotene, can even be beneficial.

Having said that, the food manufacturers, ever eager to please the customer, have been exceedingly busy over the past few years removing all kinds of additives from their products. Nowadays it's quite hard to walk down an aisle in the supermarket and find a package without the words "no artificial colors," "no artificial flavors," or "no artificial preservatives" on it. So the question of additives is gradually being taken out of our hands. But ironically, in its place, the question that food manufacturers are beginning to worry about is: How can they make the public realize that foods without preservatives just don't last as long as foods with preservatives? Food poisoning from bacteria and molds will no doubt be the hot problem of the next decade. If you choose foods without preservatives, you must remember to store them carefully according to the instructions on the package and eat them within the expiration date, which is likely to be very soon, which leads me on to . . .

THE FOOD-POISONING QUESTION

A few straightforward precautions and tips can remove most of the risk from bacteria in many everyday foods—including eggs, poultry, pre-cooked meals, and salads.

- Unless you're sure your source of eggs is salmonella-free, cook them thoroughly and avoid raw eggs, and runny poached, fried, or boiled eggs.
- Cook all meat—especially poultry—thoroughly, and scrub your hands, knives, cutting boards, and counters after handling raw meats.
- Follow cooking instructions carefully on frozen, ready-to-heat meals and pre-cooked, chilled ones. Never eat a ready-to-heat meal that is not well cooked all the way through.
- Re-wash salad greens when you get them home.
- Get your groceries home as soon as you can, preferably using an insulated bag for frozen and chilled products.
- Store raw and cooked foods separately.
- Make sure your fridge (37° F., maximum) and your freezer (0° F, maximum) are at the correct temperature.
- Don't keep cooked food for more than two days.
- Remember those most at risk from food poisoning are babies under one year old, pregnant women, the ill, and the elderly.

A SUMMARY OF WHAT YOU'VE READ IN CHAPTER 4

- You can buy all you need for a balanced, healthy diet at your favorite supermarket.
- When you shop, take a list with you.
- Don't be afraid to try all the reduced-fat items: cheeses, spreads, milk, meats, dressings, and so on.

- Try the reduced-sugar items like jams and fruits.
- Frozen, ready-to-eat meals are ideal for single dieters.
- Cans and jars are good stand-bys, and not bad for your health. Try low-calorie sauces, soups, and canned puddings.
- *Nine hundred ninety-nine people out of 1,000 will come to no harm by eating foods containing additives.*

❖ 5. ❖

Dieting Sense

Anyone can lose weight on The Junk Food Diet —safely, permanently, and healthfully. It's the simple, perfect diet for most people.

But before you even begin to read the diet itself, and most certainly before you begin to diet, it is important—no, it's *crucial*—to get yourself into the right frame of mind for losing weight. Okay, you may think you're already in the right frame of mind ("I bought the book, didn't I?" you may say. Yes, but how many others did you buy and abandon in no time?) Spend a little time here with me now, thinking about yourself and what you can do to guarantee diet success at last. You may not find that all of what follows will apply to you, but some of it will. And you have my assurance that I haven't dashed off some tips in an idle ten minutes at the end of a busy day. This little bit of dieting sense is the result of ten years' experience and observation of all kinds of people on all kinds of diets. I've been fortunate enough to have had more opportunity than any nutritionist or doctor or psychologist to study the main reasons why people fail to lose weight, even given an excellent diet, and I've had plenty of time to work out solutions, many of them tested on myself, my family, and friends!

ARE YOU FRIGHTENED OF DIETING?

I know of hundreds of people for whom the mere sound of the word *diet* is enough to produce an instant nervous headache and a sudden need to consume the complete contents of the cookie jar. Anyone who has witnessed a friend or colleague struggling through day two of his or her sixth diet this year consisting of lettuce and cottage cheese could, let's face it, be forgiven for having diet phobia and preferring to remain overweight.

So many people equate dieting with deprivation, hunger, misery, and a host of other negatives that, is it any wonder that lots of us are secretly terrified of even contemplating a diet, however badly we need and long to lose weight?

Yet, until you can conquer that fear, you'll never be able to start a diet in the right frame cf mind, let alone stick to one for more than a few days.

So let's look at the reasons for your fear.

Deprivation

Remember my promise to you—you don't have to give up the foods you like best on The Junk Food Diet. You don't have to eat foods you don't like. No Spartan regimes. No oddball ideas. So—no deprivation, right? Right.

Hunger

No. You will feel no genuine hunger on The Junk Food Diet. (I say "genuine" hunger deliberately, because many, many people who have spent months or years or all their lives eating more than they need, confuse hunger with all kinds of other feelings. There will be more on that subject later in this chapter, and more detailed help in Chapter 10.) Genuine hunger is kept at bay because we pick a dieting level for you that is right for your body, and that way you won't starve, or come anywhere near starving.

Fear of change

Diets often mean quite major changes in large chunks of our daily lives. After all, shopping, cooking, eating, drinking, and "food socializing" are a big part of most of our lives, and, especially if we lack confidence in ourselves, we enjoy familiar routines associated with food. On The Junk Food Diet I have deliberately kept any changes you will have to make to an absolute minimum. But there is another kind of change that may, secretly, frighten you. You may not even realize you're a victim of it until you read the next few paragraphs. That change is the change in yourself if the diet is a success.

The more weight you lose, the more changes you will have to accommodate. Most of these changes will be the ones you long for—to be able to wear more fashionable clothes or a swimsuit on the beach, or to be healthier, for instance. Everyone who loses weight agrees that the benefits are well worth the effort. But many people who aren't successful at losing weight are frightened—perhaps subconsciously—of the effects these changes may have on their lives. If, for example, you've spent years being everyone's "fat friend," a shoulder to cry on, you may worry that you'll lose your identity, that you'll no longer be needed. Or perhaps you've

become used to being the unattractive one, always
ignored by the opposite sex. How will it feel if you
suddenly become desirable? Or if you married your
husband or wife when you were overweight, what
will being thin do to your marriage? Will you be
tempted to have affairs? Will he/she get jealous of
your new looks? Will your friends get jealous? And
so on . . .

There aren't any easy answers to these doubts
and fears, but if some strike a chord in you, we've
probably hit upon the exact reason why you haven't
lost weight up until now. You're not so much frightened of dieting, you're frightened of being thin, of
being someone unfamiliar!

Which is why I'm going to tell you now that being
thin may make you look better, feel better, and increase your self-confidence, but it won't turn you
into someone completely different. People who genuinely love or like you now will still love or like you
when you are thin. If you lose a "friendship"
through changing your body shape, was that
"friendship" really solid or worth hanging on to by
staying fat? Equally, if you married your partner
only because he or she was the one person who
wanted you when you were fat, you may find you
want to look around again when you're thin. But if
you genuinely love your partner, you'll still be together when you've lost weight.

Fear of upsetting other people

I'm always amazed at the number of potential dieters who don't start a diet because they are frightened of upsetting family or friends—not by the
long-term results of the diet, but by short-term in-

conveniences. And it is quite astounding how selfish other people can be when it comes to your diet! If money rates as the biggest cause of marital rows, then I'm sure that diets come second. And if you have tried to cope with a diet and the tantrums and sulking that go with it, no wonder you're worried about starting another one!

So why do other people tend to react so unfavorably to your diet? All sorts of reasons. Maybe your bad temper while on previous diets has caused it. Maybe you're a diet bore, talking endlessly about calories and ounces lost. Perhaps you make everyone else feel guilty for not being on a diet, or you force everyone else to eat "rabbit food," too (husbands, especially, dread this). Last, both friends and lovers hate the wet-blanket effect that a diet often has on your social life. You won't go out for a meal or to a bar—or, if you do, you sit there sipping diet sodas.

Well, you can forget all of that hassle on The Junk Food Diet. You needn't even bother to tell friends and family that you're dieting. They'll never find out, except by looking at your shrinking poundage, of course!

Fear of failure

If you have been a habitual dieter, starting dozens but never getting beyond day two of any, you'll know only too well the guilt, and perhaps the shame, of failure. And the more often you've failed to lose weight, the more inevitable it becomes with each new dieting attempt.

Even if you say "This time I'm really going to do it," underneath you're thinking: "Why should this time be any different? In fact, why even try? Why not just admit that I'm meant to be fat and tell everyone I'm happy as I am? Or why don't I buy the diet book and say it didn't work because I have a slow metabolism?"

If fear of failure is your reason for not even trying anymore, look at it this way. Which is worse: trying one more time (but really trying this time), or being overweight, needlessly and guiltily, for the rest of your life?

I devised The Junk Food Diet for confirmed dieting failures. It doesn't induce fear, it beats it. There are no punishments for not losing a certain amount of weight in a certain time, or for a few mistakes made along the way. So go for it. You—yes, even you —can do it!

WHAT'S YOUR HURRY?

What every dieter really wants is to lose weight and never put it back on again. The most successful way of doing that is to lose slowly. The least successful way—by a mile—is to crash-diet.

So why are you in so much of a hurry to lose weight? Whether you've 10 pounds to lose or 100, losing weight too quickly is going to waste your time, not save it! Here's why.

If you haven't much weight to lose

The temptation is to follow the quickest crash diet you can find so you can get the diet out of the way and start eating normally again.

So you find your very low-calorie diet, stick it out for a week, lose your weight, and feel very pleased with yourself. "I can't be bothered messing around with slow diets," you tell your friends smugly, and you go back to your pre-crash normal diet. Within two days (yes, only two days) you've put back 3 pounds. And within another two weeks, you've put back all the weight you lost. Now you'll have to do it all over again—if and when you can be bothered to muster up the willpower to get through another week or so of deprivation. And I've got some very bad news for you. Next time it's going to be harder. There is evidence to show that people who continually lose weight, then put it back on again, also gradually replace their lean muscle tissue with more and more fat, so that each time you diet, although you may get down to your target weight, the muscle that gives your body its nice shape is decreasing, and you're getting flabbier and flabbier!

What's more, there is evidence to show that repeated diets have the cunning effect of lowering your body's metabolic rate, with the result that at the end of every new diet you can't eat as much as you used to without putting on weight again. Literally, the more you crash-diet, the less you can eat without getting fat! Horrible thought!

If you have a lot of weight to lose

Crash-dieting will give you a slightly different set of problems. First, though you may be able to stick to a very Spartan diet for a week, can you really stick to it week after week after week? If you can, you're the exception. Most people will give up and feel like failures. Then, of course, most very-low-calorie diets won't be giving you enough of all the nutrients you need, so you could be putting your health at risk with deficiencies. You could even be threatening your life by shedding lean muscle tissue (including tissue from vital organs, such as your heart) instead of fat.

Last, and probably most importantly, if you have a little or a lot to lose and you do succeed in crashing it off, you're missing the most vital role of a good diet—to help you learn how to eat in the future so that you don't put the weight back on. So, please, don't be in a hurry!

DO YOU BELIEVE IN MIRACLES?

If you're still patiently waiting for that wonderful diet miracle to come along, the one in which you eat whatever you like but still lose weight, you're not ever going to succeed on a down-to-earth, calorie-controlled diet.

It's so tempting to put your faith into an expensive magic diet pill or a cream that melts the fat away. Then, when it doesn't work, at least there's the consolation that it wasn't your fault you didn't lose weight. But in the long run, where does that get you? Certainly not any thinner. So, for anyone who is still always tempted by advertisements claiming dieting miracles of one kind or another, here is my definitive list of lotions, potions, and diet "aids" that just do not work:

- all pills that claim to slim you while you continue to eat what you like; this includes "starch blockers," said to stop all starchy foods being absorbed by your body;
- "contouring creams" that you rub into your skin;

- suits that you wear to "melt the fat away." All these suits do is help you sweat off a pint or two of liquid when you exercise. The increase in calories burned up when you wear one is minuscule;
- laxative pills, which have no effect at all on the surplus fat that is already in your body, and an adverse effect on your digestive system if taken more than occasionally.

True, you can go to your doctor, ask for, and perhaps get, one of several diet pills by prescription that may well help you to lose weight (if you can put up with the unpleasant side effects and the possibility that you will become dependent on them), but then you have the same old problem—you come off the pills and back comes the weight, which is the main reason I am totally against prescription diet pills.

So if you can't believe in miracles, what can you believe in?

Well, how about yourself? Believe in yourself and your own ability to be in full control of your own life, including your eating habits. First, think of yourself as a thin person. Think of being the size and shape you want to be. Think of buying clothes in the size you want to be and can be. Imagine yourself with the confidence to apply for a new job because your appearance is so much better than it used to be. (Don't let people convince you otherwise: Overweight people are discriminated against in the job market.)

This will all help you to stop seeing yourself as a fat person. So many overweight people tell themselves, "This is just the way I'm meant to be." The longer you've been overweight, the more inclined you are to accept the way you look as right for you. So get out of that mode of thinking. Be positive and determined that you will be thin. And don't let anyone tell you otherwise. I know many a would-be dieter who has stayed fat and "happy" for years, thanks to friends or family who insist upon saying things like, "Oh, you're lovely as you are. You're just big-boned. We're not a family of skinnies. Your face will go all gaunt if you lose weight." (You can probably think of some more.)

Of course, if you say for the twentieth time this year, "I'm going on a diet," no one will believe you. So if this is your twentieth diet, perhaps this time you would be wise to not mention it. Just get on and do it, and wait for everyone to say, "Oh, you've lost weight. Don't you look wonderful!"

I explained earlier in this chapter why some people may do anything they can to stop you from losing weight. So please don't believe them when they say you were meant to be fat. You were not. Just believe in yourself.

WHEN FOOD IS THE ENEMY

Many overweight people eat too much because food is their friend, a crutch to be turned to in times of worry, stress, boredom, or misery. Then, suddenly, when they try to diet, not only has that crutch been taken away, but food has become the enemy. Suddenly, every day seems to be one long battle.

Now, how about this for a change in thinking—enjoy your food! Enjoy tastes and textures and aromas. Accept food for what it is—enjoyable and necessary fuel for your body, the means of keeping you alive, healthy, fit, and strong. But it is not the mystical holder of special powers over you, not a substitute for friends, love, sex, hobbies, work—or anything else.

Get food back into perspective, stop battling, start relaxing and enjoying it. Then, and only then, will you become successful, thin, and an ex-fatty for life. On The Junk Food Diet you can eat any food that you want to eat, so there is no need, ever, to crave cake or freshly baked bread and feel that you aren't allowed it. Therefore, there's no need to eat the whole cake or the whole loaf, because it's always there. It's not going to run away.

HELPING YOUR DIET ALONG

Having gotten yourself into a positive frame of mind for your diet, there is still more you can do to ensure success.

Don't waste calories

Never eat a high-calorie food or drink a high-calorie drink when a low-calorie one would do just as well. For instance, if you don't mind reduced-calorie mayonnaise on your sandwiches, then don't waste calories on the regular kind. If you can take artificial sweeteners in your coffee instead of sugar, then have them. Saving calories whenever you can means that you will have some to spare for the foods you really like.

Choose the right time to begin your diet

If you're in the middle of moving, getting divorced, giving up smoking, taking exams, or have just gotten fired, this may not be the perfect time to start your diet. You are probably too preoccupied to give it your best.

Choose a time when there are no major upheavals or disappointments in your life. And a special note for women—just before your period may not be a good time to begin a diet, either, as many women retain fluid and/or feel stressed at this time of the month; wait until day five.

Get motivated

If you have some specific as well as general reasons for losing weight, you may find these help a great deal.

For instance, although it may well be enough for you to want to be healthier or to fit into smaller-sized clothes, it is much better to aim for one or two specific things: losing weight for a holiday or a wedding.

But one word of warning: If you use a specific date as your motivation, don't say something like: "By my birthday I will lose twenty-five pounds" (or whatever your ultimate target is). Simply say: "By my birthday I will lose some weight." You see, once you tell yourself you are going to lose a definite amount, if by any chance you fall short of that amount by the specified date, you will feel like a failure and probably give up, which wasn't the point of the exercise at all! And so never, ever set yourself strict goals, let alone impossible ones.

WORKING OUT HOW MUCH WEIGHT YOU WANT TO LOSE

Knowing approximately how much weight you need to lose gives you something concrete to aim for. So although you don't have a target date, you do have a target weight.

If you don't know what you should be, here are some ways of telling:

If you have ever been at your "normal" weight as an adult, what did you weigh then? You could aim for that weight again. (It's not true that you have to put on weight as you get older.)

Check the height-weight chart (Table 7, page 93). A few pounds or more above or below the average weight listed could be right for you. If in doubt, set your target at five pounds over the acceptable average listed. When you get there, you can always revise your target down a bit if you still look overweight.

What do you do if you want to lose weight and yet the height-weight chart says that you are well within the right weight for your height and frame size? Get the opinion of a sensible, unbiased friend or, failing that, a doctor or weight-loss-club adviser. If the consensus of opinion is that you don't need to lose, it could be that you simply need to do some regular exercises to tone up your body. A nonexistent waist, a protruding stomach, and flabby thighs are three areas that all respond well to a short daily toning routine that will help you look thinner, even though you weigh the same. Which brings me on to the last point . . .

SHOULD YOU EXERCISE?

If you've been a physically inactive person up to now, I think you should start building a little exercise into your day-to-day life as you lose weight. That way you burn off a few calories and you begin to realize that you have a body there that was made to do a bit of work now and then!

By exercise, though, I don't mean that you have to—or, indeed, should—take up anything really strenuous such as jogging, weight training, or squash. I was thinking more of a little daily walking.

And then I think you should try to do some body-toning exercises at least three times a week while you diet. That will help loose skin to shrink back to size and will help give you the sleek, slim look that dieting alone never quite manages to achieve, unless you are very young or very lucky. Ten to fifteen minutes a day is all you need, concentrating on you "worst" areas. Any reputable exercise book or video will help you, but don't choose an advanced program until you are advanced.

Now, all the talk is over and it's time to lose some weight!

1983 Metropolitan Height and Weight Tables*

Table 7

Height-Weight Chart for Men*

| Height | | Small | Medium | Large |
Feet	Inches	Frame	Frame	Frame
5	2	128–134	131–134	138–150
5	3	130–136	133–143	140–153
5	4	132–138	135–145	142–156
5	5	134–140	137–148	144–160
5	6	136–142	139–151	146–168
5	7	138–145	142–154	149–168
5	8	140–148	145–157	152–172
5	9	142–151	148–160	155–176
5	10	144–154	151–163	158–180
5	11	146–157	154–166	161–184
6	0	149–160	157–170	164–186
6	1	152–164	160–174	168–192
6	2	155–168	164–178	172–197
6	3	158–172	167–182	176–202
6	4	162–176	171–187	181–207

Height-Weight Chart for Women

4	10	102–111	109–121	118–131
4	11	103–113	111–123	120–134

* Weights at ages 25–59 based on lowest mortality. Weight in pounds according to frame (in indoor clothing, weight is 5 pounds for men and 3 pounds for women; shoes with 1″heels). Metropolitan Life Insurance Company Health and Safety Education Division.

Height		Small	Medium	Large
Feet	Inches	Frame	Frame	Frame
5	0	104–115	113–126	122–137
5	1	106–118	115–129	125–140
5	2	108–121	118–132	128–143
5	3	111–124	121–135	131–147
5	4	114–127	124–138	134–151
5	5	117–130	127–141	137–155
5	6	120–133	130–144	140–159
5	7	123–136	133–147	143–163
5	8	126–139	136–150	146–167
5	9	129–142	139–153	149–170
5	10	132–145	142–156	152–173
5	11	135–148	145–159	155–176
6	0	138–151	148–162	158–179

TO MAKE AN APPROXIMATION OF YOUR FRAME SIZE . . .

Extend your arm and bend the forearm upward at a 90-degree angle. Keep fingers straight and turn the inside of your wrist toward your body. Place thumb and index finger of your other hand on the two prominent bones on *either side* of your elbow. Measure the space between your fingers against a ruler or tape measure. Compare it with the following table that lists elbow measurements for medium-framed men and women. Measurements lower than those listed indicate you have a small frame. Higher measurements indicate a large frame.

Frame-Size Chart for Men

Height in 1" heels   *Elbow Breadth*

Men
5'2"–5'3"   2 1/2"–2 7/8"

5'4"–5'7"   2 5/8"–2 7/8"

5'8"–5'11"   2 3/4"–3"

6'0"–6'3"   2 3/4"–3 1/8"

6'4"   2 7/8"–3 1/4"

Frame-Size Chart for Women

Height in 1" heels   *Elbow Breadth*

Women
4'10"–4'11"   2 1/4"–2 1/2"

5'0"–5'3"   2 1/4"–2 1/2"

5'4"–5'7"   2 3/8"–2 5/8"

5'8"–5'11"   2 3/8"–2 5/8"

6'0"   2 1/2"–2 3/4"

Metropolitan Life Insurance Company Health and Safety Education Division.

A SUMMARY OF WHAT YOU'VE READ
IN CHAPTER 5

- Most people have some mental block that stops them from losing weight. Find yours for success.
- Don't be in too much of a hurry to lose weight. The only way to diet and *never* put the weight back on is to lose slowly.
- Believe in yourself, not in dieting miracles.
- Food isn't your best friend or your deadly enemy. Learn to relax around it.
- Help your diet help you.
- Get some exercise.

❖ 6. ❖

The Junk Food Diet—1

PICK THE PLAN FOR YOU!

THE JUNK FOOD DIET BEGINS RIGHT HERE! AND THE first thing we must do is ensure that you'll be eating the right amount for you while on it—an essential that many diets forget.

A physically active girl of twenty-one, for instance, will need many more calories a day when she's dieting than a fifty-year-old inactive woman, even if they both want to lose the same amount of weight. And, conversely, two thirty-year-old men of the same height will probably have different calorie requirements, depending on how much they want to lose and what exercise they do. That's why, with the help of my special dieter's questionnaire that follows, we find the perfect plan for you. And that's why anyone can lose weight on The Junk Food Diet.

The diet itself, no matter how many calories a day you are on, is in two stages. First there's a Set Diet, lasting a minimum of two weeks. You'll start on approximately 1,000, 1,250 or 1,500 calories a day, depending upon your answers to the questionnaire. Then, if you have more weight to lose, you either stay on your Set Diet or, if you prefer, you move to the Pick Your Own Plan, an ultra-flexible diet that allows you maximum control over what you eat, when you eat, how you eat, and where you eat. I have simply taken all the hard work out of dieting for you on this plan (as you'll discover in Chapter 8) until you're right down to your target weight.

FINDING YOUR CALORIE LEVEL

Following are eight crucial questions, with a different score for each answer. All you have to do is pick one answer to each question and write the appropriate score in the box at the end of each line. When you've answered all the questions, add up your score and check what it means. (Do be honest with yourself about the answers to questions 5 through 8, because bending the truth will only result in your getting the wrong score, and perhaps the wrong diet!)

Questionnaire

	Available score	*Your score*
1. Your sex:		
Male	5	
Female	1	
2. Your age:		
21 or under	4	
22–30	3	
31–50	2	
51 or over	1	

	Available score	Your score

3. Your height:

	Available score	Your score
Over 5′11″	4	
5′6½″–5′11″	3	
5′2½″–5′6″	2	
5′2″ or under	1	

4. Amount of weight you need to lose*:

	Available score	Your score
Over 45 pounds	5	
15 to 45 pounds	3	
15 to 30 pounds	2	
15 pounds or less	1	

5. Your working/regular day is:

	Available score	Your score
Very physically active—spend most of time on the move (*e.g.*, sports teacher, builder)	3	
Fairly physically active—spend several hours a day on feet (*e.g.*, sales person, postman)	2	
Sedentary—spend less than one hour a day on the move (*e.g.*, word-processor operator, receptionist)	1	

* See page 91 in Chapter 5 if you need help on this.

	Available score	*Your score*

6. Amount of exercise (over and above that covered by question 5):

Regular—at least three times a week sustained —at least 30 minutes a time—aerobic activity *(e.g.,* jogging, swimming, cycling) — 3 — ☐

Regular sustained mild aerobic activity *(e.g.,* walking) — 2 — ☐

Little or no regular sustained exercise — 1 — ☐

7. Dieting history—choose whichever of the following statements is closest to your experience:

Haven't dieted at all in recent years — 3 — ☐

Often start diets, lose a little, give up, never get down to target weight — 2 — ☐

Have gotten down to target weight at least once, but always put it back on again — 1 — ☐

Have been losing weight recently on another diet — 1 — ☐

	Available score	Your score

8. Choose whichever of the
   following statements
   most closely matches
   your ideal diet:

   I prefer to lose weight very
   slowly if it means I can
   eat a little more   3

   I would like to lose weight
   steadily   2

   I would like to lose weight
   as fast as safely possible   1

Check your score:

8–12
Your Set Diet is Diet One (approximately 1,000 calories a day); see page 115.

13–20
Your Set Diet is Diet Two (approximately 1,250 calories a day); see page 126.

21–30
Your Set Diet is Diet Three (approximately 1,500 calories a day); see page 137.

YOUR SET DIET

One each of the three Set Diets, every day's eating for a minimum of 14 days, is specified. There is still plenty of choice, though, to ensure that you will be eating the way you like to eat. This diet will get your dieting off to a great start because:

* It is easy to follow.
* When you're starting a diet, a set format helps bolster your determination.
* It gives you a sense of security.
* It shows you exactly what a varied diet is like, so if (and when) you switch to the Pick Your Own Plan, or a maintenance plan, you'll be better equipped.

When you have been on the Set Diet for a minimum of two weeks, you have a choice of action.

If you don't need to lose any more weight, turn to Chapter 11 and find out how to keep that weight off!

If you do need to lose more weight, you can either continue with your Set Diet by returning to the beginning of it and repeating the 14 days, or you can move to the Pick Your Own Plan. The choice is yours, but if you have more than 15 pounds left to lose, I do recommend that you move to the Pick Your Own Plan, as it offers much more flexibility— you create your own diet without having to do anything other than select a menu geared to your personal calorie total, and there is the added bonus of "eating out" and "days off" schemes built in!

Even if you are on the Pick Your Own Plan, you can return to the Set Diet any time you like. You'll find more information about both Set Diets and

Pick Your Own Plans at the start of chapters 7 and 8.

What to expect when you start dieting

When you begin your diet, here's what will happen. The 14-day Set Diet could see you lose from 7 pounds up to as much as 15 pounds, depending on your starting weight (the more you need to lose and the taller you are, the greater your initial weight loss will be) and other personal factors.

In the first week, the loss will be largest of all, and the reason is that when you first reduce your calorie intake, your body uses up its carbohydrate store and loses surplus water, too. After a few more days of dieting, the fluid loss will stop and any more weight you lose will be mostly fat. So, in the second week, your weight loss will be smaller.

This is normal and correct, and not because the diet "isn't working" or because you've done anything wrong. It is what happens to everyone.

As your diet progresses

When you've been dieting for a while longer, you'll probably notice that you don't lose exactly the same amount every week, however carefully you have been sticking to your diet. This isn't anything to worry about, either. For women, in particular, weight-loss fluctuation can be quite spectacular. Often in the first two weeks of their menstrual cycle, they lose a lot; in mid-cycle they lose a steady amount; and just before a period they may put weight on, no matter how carefully they've dieted.

This weight gain is fluid, not fat, and it will disappear around the third day of the period.

Weight-loss fluctuations from week to week, whatever your sex, don't really matter. What does matter is that over the course of, say, a month, you weigh less than you did the previous month. If over the course of a whole month, however, you don't lose a single pound (assuming you're not at your target weight yet, of course!) read on. . . .

If your weight loss slows down immediately or stops

The nearer you get to your target weight, the more likely you are to find your weight loss slowing down. This doesn't necessarily mean that you have been cheating. There is a scientific explanation. As you lose weight you need fewer calories (that's why a 110-pound girl needs to eat less than a 210-pound man). So, if, for instance, you now weigh 140 pounds instead of your previous 180 pounds, you will need to eat less to maintain your new weight, and less on your weight-loss diet to keep up a suitable calorie deficit—unless you increase your exercise.

This "sticking point" or "plateau" often happens about two-thirds of the way down toward your target weight. Your weight loss might slow down from, say, two pounds a week to half a pound a week, and then it stops altogether. Of course, everyone is different and your plateau might be reached earlier, or later, or even not at all. It is certainly not going to happen while you are on your first 14-day Set Diet. But when it does happen, you can increase your body's calorie needs by stepping up your activity. You could burn up an extra 100 calories with, for example, a half-hour medium-paced walk, a fifteen-minute cycle ride, or a ten-minute jog. It's healthier to increase your exercise than to reduce your calories.

Ninety-nine percent of dieters need never go below 1,000 calories a day to reach their target weight, 50 percent will never have to go below 1,250, and many will reach their target weight still on 1,500. So don't worry about reaching a plateau until it happens.

And if it does, here's one other small thought. You've been on your diet for a while. Are you checking your portion sizes? In other words, is that 1/4 cup of mashed potatoes really 1/4 cup, or is it a 1/2 cup? Is that teaspoon of butter nearer a tablespoon? You need only a couple of portion mistakes on the generous side each day to tip the balance from steady weight loss to little or no weight loss. This is the most likely explanation of your problem if weight loss is very slow early on in your diet rather than toward the end. So before you do anything else, check it out.

If you lose weight too quickly

The calorie level we've chosen for you should result in a steady weight loss of anything up to 3 pounds a week. But there are always exceptions to the rule. If, after the initial week's big weight loss, you are losing more than this, you might think about increasing your calorie level. The main problem with losing weight too quickly (discussed in more detail in Chapter 5) is that you may get hungry and give up your diet. So if you are losing weight quickly and feel hungry—especially if you were a borderline case in our questionnaire—step up to the next calorie rank. Already on 1,500? A few people—mostly active men and teen-agers, or people with a lot of weight to lose—may find they can diet successfully on 1,600 calories, or even more, a day. If that happens to you, simply add 100 calories a day to your diet from the Pick Your Own Snack listings on pages 197–202.

TIPS

The following dieting tips apply to everyone throughout their weight-loss program.

- Plan your day's eating well in advance when possible.
- Keep a diary and record of how much you've eaten, what you ate, what you liked, your thoughts, etc. It helps.
- Drink plenty of calorie-free drinks; they help fill you up and keep your digestive system working well (for a list, see page 108.)
- Eat everything you are allowed on your diet.
- Take your time over your food; research shows that thin people eat more slowly!

RULES

Following are mandatory rules to help you get the most benefit from your diet! They also apply to everyone throughout the diet.

- Weigh yourself no more than once a week.
- Vary your meal choices as much as possible, aiming not to have the same main meal more than once a week.

- When cooking red meats, bacon, etc., cook until well done enough for most of the fat to run out. If making gravy or sauces, pour off or skim away fat first.

- When frying use a non-stick pan and ensure that oil is at the correct, high temperature before adding food. Fry in corn, sunflower, safflower, rapeseed, or olive oil; don't use lard. Drain food well on paper towels.

- Remove visible fat and skin from meat before cooking.

- Eat when you're hungry, not by the clock. If you ever get hungry between or after meals, and you don't have any snacks to spare, choose items from the Unlimiteds list (direction).

- Weigh or measure foods when amounts are stated.

- Don't waste calories. Never use a high-calorie ingredient in cooking or preparing food when a lower-calorie one would do just as well, and never eat anything you don't really want or need.

- If you have a day—or more—when your dieting gets off course, for whatever reason, don't let it tempt you to give up. For more detailed advice on coping with dieting disasters and problems, turn to chapters 9 and 10.

Guidelines for Sweet-Toothers

If you are choosing your "treats" calorie allowance in sweet items, follow these rules:

- Never eat your sweet treats when you are really hungry. Always satisfy hunger first, with a sa-

vory food snack or meal within your diet. Then
have the sweet food.

- It is better to choose a single-item sweet food,
  such as a slice of cake or a chocolate bar, and eat
  it all at once than pick a pack of mints or candies
  that will stay in your mouth over a long period.
- It is better to eat your sweet treat as part of a
  meal—say, as a dessert—than on its own.
- Brush your teeth after each sweet treat.
- Never go to bed at night without brushing and
  flossing teeth thoroughly.

UNLIMITEDS

Quantities of all the following foods, drinks, and
seasonings are unlimited throughout your diet.
That means that you can have them whenever you
like, in reasonable amounts. The Eats will help fill
you up, add color and variety to your diet, and help
provide vital nutrients. The Drinks will also help
fill you up and help your digestive system. The Others will add taste and variety to your diet. However,
none of the Unlimiteds is mandatory—with the obvious exception of your own choice of drinks, without which you would soon die!—so if you choose not
to have them, you will still get a healthy, balanced,
varied diet from the basic Junk Food Diet presented
in the following chapters.

Drinks

Water, mineral water, soda water, calorie-free
mixes and canned sodas, calorie-free iced teas and
coffee, black tea, black coffee, herbal tea.

Eats

Lettuce, tomato, watercress, onion, cucumber, cabbage, Chinese cabbage, cauliflower, greens, green beans, zucchini, carrots, celery, peppers, radishes, bean sprouts, mushrooms. All these can be raw or cooked without fat.

Others

Fresh or dried herbs and spices, oil-free salad dressing, lemon juice, Worcestershire sauce, soy sauce, mustard, garlic, vinegar, lemon slices.

The Junk Food Diet—2

THE SET DIETS

BEFORE YOU BEGIN THE SET DIET THAT WE DECIDED was right for you in the last chapter, read through the following notes.

Breakfast

Every day there is a choice of two breakfasts. If you don't like breakfast at "breakfast time," you can eat this meal anytime during the day as an extra snack. In fact, if you habitually don't eat breakfast, I strongly advise you not to start trying now. As least one of the breakfasts every day can be packed, so you could perhaps take it to work and eat it as a mid-morning snack.

Light meal

Most people will want to eat this around lunchtime, but if you happen to prefer your main meal at lunchtime, this will be your supper. There is a choice of either a hot, light meal or a cold one, which can be packed for a working lunch—or you could eat it in the park, or in the cafeteria, while you talk with friends.

Main meal

There are four choices of main meal: a family choice
of a recipe dish; a quick and easy meal suitable for
singles, non-cooks, and people in a hurry; the heat-
and-serve alternative, which is a complete ready
meal, usually with the addition of a vegetable or
salad; and, last, there is a takeout choice.

Snacks

Every day you choose two Snacks. One is a choice of
either milk (which you can use in drinks or as a
drink on its own) or yogurt; the other is fruit.

The milk Snack on all diets is 3/4 cup skim milk,
which can be used either in your tea or coffee or as a
drink on its own. If you prefer your drinks black
and don't like drinking milk, have a low-calorie diet
fruit yogurt, such as Weight Watchers, instead. (Ordinary fruit yogurts marked "low fat" aren't particularly low in calories; look for a brand that is
around 50 calories a container.)

The fruit Snack is one of the following fruits every day: 1 apple, 2 apricots, 1/2 cup cherries, 1/2 cup
unsweetened fruit salad, 1/2 cup grapes, 1 small
grapefruit, 2 small plums, 1 tangerine, 1/4 cantaloupe, 1/6 honeydew, 1 nectarine, 1 orange, 1/2 pa-
paya, 1 pear, 2 pineapple rings, 1/2 cup any soft
berry *(e.g.,* raspberries, strawberries, or blackberries), 1/2 cup any stewed fruit *(e.g.,* apple or rhubarb,
cooked either with sugar from your treats list, or
sweetened with artificial sweetener).

Your fruits should be fresh, if possible, or frozen,
as a good alternative. If you use canned fruits now
and then, drain them of the syrup or juice and

weigh them or measure them out then. If for any reason one day you can't get your fruit supply, have instead 1/2 cup of fruit juice or 1 ounce of dried apricots or raisins—that's about 4 pieces of dried fruit, or 1/4 cup of raisins.

Treats/Extras

Every day you can choose a Treat or an Extra: 100, 150 or 250 calories' worth a day, depending on which diet level you are on.

Treats can be either sweet—such as cake, cookies desserts and chocolate—or alcohol, or savory things, such as bread and butter, or chips, instead. They can be eaten as a dessert or as a snack whenever you like during the day. If you're choosing sweet Treats, follow the tips on page 107 in Chapter 6.

Instead of a Treat, you could choose an Extra: an addition to your meal, for instance, such as extra fries, rice, or mayonnaise, or butter on your baked potato. It's up to you how you spend this Treats allowance. Full lists of the allowed Treats and Extras appear on pages 197–202.

Unlimiteds

Don't forget to make the most of your Unlimiteds—the foods and drinks listed in Chapter 6 that will help broaden your diet's horizons.

The Sunday brunch alternative

There are two sorts of Sunday eaters: those who have a light breakfast, a big lunch (probably a traditional one), and a supper; and those who have a late, combined breakfast/lunch, then a main meal in the evening. Decide which pattern you prefer and follow the appropriate Sunday diet.

Salad

Salad items are mentioned as accompaniments with some light and main meals. If you don't like the items mentioned, pick an alternative from the Unlimiteds list. When simply "salad" is mentioned, choose whatever you like from the list in whatever quantity. If you're a total salad-hater and follow the diet without any of these items, make doubly sure to eat all fruit and fruit juice allowed on the diet and get your full quota of vegetables mentioned. If you choose takeout frequently, this advice is even more important.

Milk

Your daily snack and cereal milk should be skim, but if you refuse to drink skim milk, low fat or 1% fat will add only an extra 20 to 30 calories a day to your diet. Whole milk is a terrible waste of calories, in my opinion, but if you must have it, you can choose it as all or part of your daily Treat/Extra.

Frying

Here are some notes on the frying methods used in The Junk Food Diet.

- Dry-frying: Use a good, heavy, non-stick pan. Wipe the bottom with a smear of oil on a paper towel or a two-second spray with a vegetable

cooking spray. Heat the pan. With eggs, add them
to a hot pan. With fatty meat such as bacon, add
to a warm pan and gradually increase the heat
until the fat runs out and the bacon (or whatever)
cooks in its own fat. Always drain off any fat left
in the pan at the end of cooking and pat the food
dry on paper towels.

- Stir-frying: Use a good non-stick pan or wok. Add
one or two teaspoons of oil and turn heat up high.
Add shredded or stripped vegetables, meat, etc.,
as instructed, and stir constantly until food is just
cooked. Add stock or water, not extra oil, if food
gets too dry.

- Shallow- or deep-frying: Make sure the oil is very
hot before adding the food. Don't over-fry. Remove food on a slotted spatula or spoon and place
on paper towels and drain thoroughly. Never
refry fried foods to reheat them. They'll absorb
twice as much fat.

- French fries: Whenever oven fries are mentioned
in the diet, you could substitute very thick-cut,
deep-fried fries instead—*e.g.,* steak fries or homemade fries.

Finally . . .

Start the diet on a Monday. Make sure you have
everything you need beforehand. Don't swap
around meals from different days.

DIET ONE

(approximately 1,000 calories a day)

Every day:
  You may have Unlimiteds from the list on page 108.

  You should have your two Snacks—your milk or yogurt and your fruit.

  You can pick Treats/Extras up to 100 calories a day from the list on pages 197–202.

Day 1

Breakfast
Either 1 medium slice bread with 1 teaspoon diet margarine and 2 teaspoons of reduced-sugar jam or jelly, 1 diet fruit yogurt, 1/2 cup unsweetened orange, grapefruit, or pineapple juice;

or 1 ounce breakfast cereal of choice with 1/2 cup milk and 1 teaspoon sugar, 1/2 cup unsweetened orange, grapefruit, or low-calorie cranberry juice.

Light meal
Either 1 Le Menu Light Style Glazed Chicken Breast, 1 tomato;

or 1 Lean Cuisine Chicken and Vegetables with Vermicelli;

or 3 Rye Krisps or 1 mini pita pocket, filled with a mixture of 3 ounces cold cooked chicken or turkey, chopped, 1 level tablespoon reduced-calorie mayonnaise, chopped tomato and green pepper, 1 tablespoon diced onion, 1 apple.

Main meal

Family Choice: 1 serving Chili Con Carne (see recipe, page 285) with small green salad.

Quick and Easy: 1 beef frankfurter—well grilled or
fried;

or 1 pork chop, trimmed, 1/4 cup baked beans, and
1/4 cup instant mashed potatoes or 2 ounces oven
fries, baked.

Heat and Serve: 1 8-ounce can Heinz Baked Beans
with Franks, 1 medium slice bread with a little imitation diet margarine.

Takeout: **Either** 1 Wendy's Baked Potato with Chili
and Cheese;

or 1 Taco Bell Double Beef Burrito.

Day 2

Breakfast

Either 2 medium slices bread with a little imitation
diet margarine and 3 teaspoons reduced-sugar jam
or marmalade, 1/2 grapefruit or 4 ounces canned
grapefruit segments;

or shredded wheat, 1 teaspoon sugar, 1/2 cup milk,
1/2 grapefruit or 4 ounces canned grapefruit segments.

Light meal

Either 1 medium egg, dry-fried, 3 ounces oven
chips;

or 2 medium eggs, scrambled, on 1 medium slice
toast;

or 2 medium slices bread, 1 medium egg, hard-
boiled, 1 teaspoon reduced-calorie mayonnaise,
sliced tomato and lettuce leaves.

Main meal

Family Choice: 1 portion Beef Stir-Fry (see recipe, page 289, 1/2 cup mixed peas and carrots.

Quick and Easy: 1 beef burger, dry-fried, 3 ounces oven chips or 1/4 cup instant mashed potatoes, 1 tomato.

Heat and Serve: **Either** 1 Banquet Pot Pie, small salad with 1 teaspoon reduced-calorie dressing;
or Swanson Beef in Barbeque Sauce, small salad with 1 teaspoon reduced-calorie dressing.

Takeout: **Either** 1 McDonald's Quarterpounder without cheese;
or 1 Jack In The Box Hot Club Supreme.

Day 3

Breakfast

Either 1 medium slice bread with one teaspoon diet margarine, 1 boiled egg, 1/2 unsweetened orange, grapefruit, or pineapple juice;
or 1 medium slice bread with one teaspoon diet margarine and 2 teaspoons reduced-sugar jam or marmalade, 1 banana.

Light meal

Either 1 large hot dog, heated, in 1 hot dog roll with 2 tablespoons onion slices and ketchup or mustard of choice;
or 2 medium slices toast or 4 Rye Krisps, 2 ounces (1/4 can) tuna salad, lettuce and tomato, 2 ounces Lite Line cheese.

Main meal
Family Choice: 1 portion Macaroni and Cheese (see recipe, page 278), 1/2 cup green beans, or small salad.
Quick and Easy: 1 grilled cheese-and-tomato sandwich made with vegetable cooking spray, 1/3 cup green beans, 1 tomato.
Heat and Serve: **Either** 1 Lean Cuisine Lasagna; **or** 1 Weight Watchers Pasta Primavera, both with 1/3 cup green beans or large side salad.
Takeout: 2 slices Pizza Hut Thin-n Crispy Cheese Pizza.

Day 4

Breakfast
Same as Day 1.

Light meal
Either 8-ounce baked potato with 2 tablespoons grated cheese;
or 2 thin slices toast, 2 ounces lean ham with mustard, 1 small tomato, sliced.

Main meal
Family Choice: **Either** 1 portion Beef Goulash (see recipe, page 287), 1/2 cup boiled rice or noodles, 1/3 cup peas;
or 1 portion Marinated Ginger Pork (see recipe, page 292), 1/3 cup boiled rice or noodles, 1/3 cup cooked peas.
Quick and Easy: 4-ounce hamburger, well grilled or broiled and well drained, 1/3 cup boiled rice or noodles, 1/3 cup peas.

Heat and Serve: **Either** Le Menu Beef Burgundy, side salad with oil-free dressing;
or 1 Armour Beef Stroganoff, side salad with oil-free dressing.
Takeout: Same as day 2.

Day 5

Breakfast
Same as Day 2.

Light meal
Either 2 medium eggs made into omelet, cooked in non-stick pan, 1 slice whole-wheat toast, 1 tomato;
or 1 small pita bread with 2 hard-cooked eggs with 2 teaspoons reduced-calorie mayonnaise.

Main meal
Family Choice: 1 portion Fisherman's Soup (see recipe, page 267), chilled broccoli spears with reduced-calorie dressing, 1 roll with 1 teaspoon reduced-calorie margarine;
Quick and Easy: **Either** 6-ounce fillet of white fish with 1 portion Cheese Sauce (see recipe page 259), 1/4 cup instant mashed potatoes, 1/4 cup sweet corn or peas;
or 4 fish sticks, baked, 1/4 cup instant mashed potatoes, 1/4 cup peas or baked beans.
Heat and Serve: 1 Mrs. Paul's Fish Au Gratin, 2 broccoli spears or 1/4 cup green beans or mixed salad.
Takeout: **Either** 1 McDonald's Filet-O-Fish;
or 1 Jack In The Box Fish Supreme (no Treats allowed today if you choose takeout).

Day 6

Breakfast
Either 3 slices crisp bacon, 1 slice toast, 1/2 cup unsweetened orange, grapefruit, or pineapple juice;
or 1 thin slice bread with 1 teaspoon diet margarine
and 1 teaspoon reduced-sugar jam, 1 shredded-
wheat biscuit with 1/2 cup skim milk.

Light meal
Either 5-inch cheese-and-tomato pizza, grilled,
mixed salad;
or 2 ounces reduced-fat Cheddar-style cheese with 5
saltine crackers or 3-inch piece French bread with a
little mustard, side salad with oil-free dressing.

Main meal
Family Choice: **Either** 1 portion Tandoori Chicken
(see recipe, page 272), with 1/2 cup boiled rice, sliced
tomato salad;
or 1 portion Chicken and Broccoli Casserole (see
recipe, page 274), 1/2 cup green beans.
Quick and Easy: 1 average chicken breast half without skin, boiled or baked, 1 small baked potato, 1/3
cup sweet corn or peas.
Heat and Serve: 1 Lean Cuisine Chicken Cacciatore
with Vermicelli.
Takeout: **Either** 1 portion chicken chow mein;
or 1 Roy Rogers Fried Chicken Breast, cole slaw (no
Treats allowed today if you choose either of these
takeouts).

Day 7

Breakfast
Either 1 medium poached egg, 2 slices bread, 2 teaspoons reduced-sugar jelly, 1/2 cup orange juice;
or 2 ounces crisply cooked lean bacon or ham, 1
slice whole-wheat toast, 1/2 cup milk, 1/2 cantaloupe.

Light meal
Either 1 10-ounce can pea soup, 1 slice bread;
or 1/8 of a 9-inch quiche, side salad with oil-free
dressing.

Main meal
Family Choice: 3 ounces well-done lean roast beef or
leg of lamb or loin of pork, 1 small baked or boiled
potato, 1/2 cup broccoli or green beans or cauliflower, 1/2 cup carrots, 1 small piece fresh fruit of
choice.
Quick and Easy: 4-ounce beefburger, broiled, 3
ounces oven fries or 1 burger bun, 1/4 cup sweet corn
or side salad, ketchup or mustard.
Heat and Serve: 1 Swanson Hungry-Man Sliced
Beef.
Takeout: **Either** 1 roast beef sandwich;
or 1 Taco Bell Beef Burrito.

Sunday brunch exchange
If you prefer, have the following brunch instead of
both the Day 7 breakfast and the light meal (so you
have just a brunch and a main meal today): 1/2 cantaloupe or 1/4 honeydew or 1 cup orange juice, 2
medium eggs, dry-fried, 1 breakfast sausage link,
well fried or broiled, 1 potato pancake, dry-fried, or

1/2 cup home fries, 1 slice bacon, well grilled, 1 medium slice bread with a little diet margarine.

Day 8

Breakfast
Same as Day 1.

Light meal
Either 3 ounces leftover roast meat, 1/4 cup oven fries, 1 tomato, sliced, with oil-free dressing;
or 2 medium slices bread with a little mustard, 2 ounces cold roast meat, lettuce leaves.

Main meal
Family Choice: 4 ounces lean boiled ham, 1 small potato, 1/3 cup green peas or 2/3 cup broccoli.
Quick and Easy: 4-ounce ham steak, broiled, 1/4 cup instant mashed potatoes, 1/3 cup peas or corn.
Heat and Serve: 1 Armour Ham Steak Dinner, salad.
Takeout: 1 ham-and-swiss sandwich on rye bread.

Day 9

Breakfast
Same as Day 2.

Light meal
Either 1 flounder fillet, broiled, 1/4 cup instant mashed potatoes, 1/2 cup green beans;
or 2 medium slices bread, 1 31/2-ounce can tuna in water, drained, lettuce leaves, 2 teaspoons reduced-calorie dressing.

Main meal
Family Choice: **Either** 1 portion Turkey Meat Loaf
(see recipe, page 273) 1 small potato or 1/2 cup rice,
1/2 cup peas;
or 1 portion Beef Stroganoff (see recipe, page 288),
1/2 cup boiled noodles.
Quick and Easy: 1 La Choy Sweet and Sour Pork,
side salad with reduced-calorie dressing.
Heat and Serve: 1 Le Menu Yankee Pot Roast Dinner.
Takeout: Taco Bell Beef Burrito, side salad without
dressing.

Day 10

Breakfast
Same as Day 3.

Light meal
Either 1 medium egg, dry-fried, 2 slices bacon, well
cooked until crisp, 2 slices bread, 1 tomato;
or 2 slices bread with 1 teaspoon reduced-calorie
mayonnaise, 2 slices very lean ham, lettuce and
sliced tomato, 1 teaspoon mustard.

Main meal
Family Choice: **Either** 1 portion Risotto (see recipe,
page 283), side salad with oil-free dressing;
or 1 portion Shrimp Provençale (see recipe, page
268), 1/2 cup boiled rice, side salad with oil-free
dressing.
Quick and Easy: broiled 1/2 chicken breast without
skin, 1/4 cup instant mashed potatoes, 1/2 cup corn.
Heat and Serve: **Either** 1 Gorton's Shrimp Scampi;
or 1 Budget Gourmet Scallop and Shrimp Mariner

with Rice, both with salad with reduced-calorie dressing.
Takeout: **Either** 1 Burger King Whaler Sandwich*;
or McDonald's Filet-O-Fish*;
or 1 Jack In The Box Pasta Seafood Salad.

Day 11

Breakfast
Same as Day 4.

Light meal
Either 2 ounces reduced-fat cheese, melted on 1 medium slice toast, topped with sliced tomato;
or 2 mini pitas or 1 large pita filled with 2 tablespoons low-fat cream cheese, chopped vegetables of choice *(e.g.,* peppers, tomato, onion), 2 black olives.

Main meal
Family Choice: **Either** 1 portion Beef Goulash (see recipe, page 287);
or 1 portion Beef Stroganoff (see recipe, page 288), both with 1/4 cup boiled rice, 1/3 cup peas or 1/2 cup broccoli.
Quick and Easy: 4-ounce beefburger, broiled, 3 ounces oven fries, 1 tomato, broiled.
Heat and Serve: 1 Le Menu Beef Burgundy, side salad with reduced-calorie dressing.
Takeout: 1/4 order of Chinese beef and green peppers with oyster sauce, 1 cup plain rice (no Treats allowed today if you choose this takeout).

---

* No Treats allowed today if you choose this takeout.

Day 12

Breakfast
Same as Day 5.

Light meal
Either 1 10-ounce can Campbell's Chunky Chicken Soup, 1 medium roll, 1 teaspoon diet margarine; **or** 2 slices bread with 1 teaspoon reduced-calorie mayonnaise, 2 lean slices chicken or turkey or ham, 2 lettuce leaves, mustard.

Main meal
Family Choice: **Either** 1 portion Cod Creole (see recipe, page 269), 1/2 cup peas, 1/2 cup boiled rice; **or** 1 portion Tuna Florentine (see recipe, page 266).
Quick and Easy: 1 haddock or cod fillet (frozen) in light and crispy batter, baked; 3 ounces oven chips, 1/3 cup peas.
Heat and Serve: 1 Lean Cuisine Linguine with Clam Sauce, side salad with oil-free dressing, 1 small roll.
Takeout: 2 slices cheese pizza.

Day 13

Breakfast
Same as Day 6.

Light meal
Either 1 Chef Boyardee Microwave Bowl Lasagna, 1 small roll; **or** 2 ounces Brie cheese, 4 crackers or crispbreads, salad with oil-free dressing.

Main meal

Family Choice: 4 ounces lean roast chicken or turkey, 1 small boiled potato, 2 large broccoli spears, 1/3 cup stuffing.

Quick and Easy: 1 chicken breast without skin, hot or cold; 1/2 cup potato salad, green salad with oil-free dressing.

Heat and Serve: 1 Swanson Sweet and Sour Chicken, side salad with oil-free dressing.

Takeout: 1 Kentucky Fried Chicken Breast, baked beans, coleslaw.

Sunday brunch exchange

Same as Day 7.

DIET TWO

(approximately 1,250 calories a day)

Every day:

You may have Unlimiteds from the list on page 108.

You should have two Snacks—your milk or yogurt, and your fruit.

You can pick Treats/Extras up to 150 calories a day from the lists on pages 197–202.

Day 1

Breakfast

Either 1 medium slice bread with 2 teaspoons reduced-sugar jam or jelly, 1 diet yogurt, 1/2 cup unsweetened orange juice;

or 1 ounce breakfast cereal of choice with 1 cup

milk and 1 teaspoon sugar, 1/2 cup unsweetened orange, grapefruit, or pineapple juice.

Light meal

Either 2 ounces chicken or turkey meat, 2 slices bread with 2 teaspoons reduced-calorie mayonnaise, mustard, lettuce, and tomato;
or 1 small cooked chicken breast or 3 ounces leftover chicken meat, 1 large salad with reduced-calorie dressing, 1 thin slice bread.

Main meal

Family Choice: 1 serving Turkey Meat Loaf (see recipe, page 273) 1/4 cup instant mashed potatoes, 1/2 cup green beans.
Quick and Easy: 1 jumbo beef hot dog, 1/4 cup instant mashed potatoes, 1/2 cup baked beans.
Heat and Serve: Swanson Beans with Franks Dinner.
Takeout: Hot dog with cheese, 1 small order french fries.

Day 2

Breakfast

Either 2 medium slices bread with 2 tablespoons reduced-sugar jam or marmalade, 1/2 grapefruit or 1/2 cup canned grapefruit segments;
or 2 shredded-wheat biscuits, 1 teaspoon sugar, 1 cup milk, 1/2 grapefruit or 1/2 cup canned grapefruit segments.

Light meal

Either 3 ounces reduced-fat American cheese, melted on 1 slice toast topped with 1 sliced tomato;

or 3 ounces reduced-fat American cheese with 1 medium slice bread or 4 crackers, a little mustard, 1 tomato, 1 medium apple.

Main meal

Family Choice: 1 serving Beef Goulash (see recipe, page 287), 1/2 cup green beans.

Quick and Easy: 3 ounces sliced lean roast beef, 1/2 cup beets, 1/2 cup potato salad, side salad with oil-free dressing.

Heat and Serve: 1 Le Menu Beef Sirloin Tips, sliced tomato salad with oil-free dressing.

Takeout: **Either** McDonald's Quarterpounder without cheese;

or 1 Roy Rogers Roast Beef Sandwich, 1 regular order potato salad.

Day 3

Breakfast

Either 1 medium slice bread with 1 teaspoon diet margarine, 1 hard-cooked egg, 1/2 cup unsweetened orange, grapefruit, or pineapple juice;

or 1 medium slice bread with 1 teaspoon diet margarine, 2 teaspoons reduced-sugar jam or marmalade, 1/2 banana or 1 container diet yogurt.

Light meal

Either 1 single-serving can Campbell's Chunky Minestrone Soup or 1 single-serving can Campbell's Chunky Chicken and Rice Soup, 1 slice bread;

or 3 ounces very lean ham, 2 slices bread with 1 tablespoon reduced-calorie mayonnaise, 1 sliced tomato.

Main meal
Family Choice: 1 portion Potato Frittata (see recipe, page 265), 1/2 cup peas.
Quick and Easy: 2 medium eggs, dry-fried, 4 ounces oven chips, 1/2 cup peas, 1 apple.
Heat and Serve: 1 Swanson Great Starts Omelette with Sausage and Cheese, side salad, 1/4 cup corn.
Takeout: 1 Burger King Scrambled Egg Platter.

Day 4

Breakfast
Same as Day 1.

Light meal
1 3 1/2-ounce can tuna in water, drained, 1 average bread roll or 2 small slices bread with 2 teaspoons reduced-calorie mayonnaise, lettuce.

Main meal
Family Choice: 1 portion Vegetable Lasagna Rolls (see recipe, page 282), side salad with oil-free dressing.
Quick and Easy: 4-ounce beefburger, broiled, 3 ounces oven fries, 1/4 cup peas or corn or baked beans.
Heat and Serve: **Either** 1 Swanson Spaghetti with Meatballs with 2 tablespoons Parmesan cheese;
or 1 Stouffer's Lasagna with 2 tablespoons Parmesan cheese.
Takeout: 3 slices Pizza Hut Thin-n Crispy Cheese Pizza.

Day 5

Breakfast
Same as day 2.

Light meal
Either 2 medium eggs, poached or scrambled with 1
tablespoon diet margarine on 1 medium slice toast;
or 1 hard-cooked egg with large salad, 1 tablespoon
reduced-calorie mayonnaise.

Main meal
Family Choice: 1 serving Fish Kebabs (see recipe,
page 270), 1/2 cup boiled rice, side salad with oil-free
dressing.
Quick and Easy: 1 Gorton's Light Recipe Lightly
Breaded Fish Fillets, 1/4 cup instant mashed pota-
toes, 1/3 cup peas or baked beans, 1 banana.
Heat and Serve: Gorton's Seafood Lover's Fillets Al-
mondine, side salad with oil-free dressing.
Takeout: 1 McDonald's Filet-O-Fish.

Day 6

Breakfast
Either 3 slices crisp bacon on 1 medium slice toast,
1/2 cup unsweetened orange, grapefruit, or pineapple juice;
or 1 small slice bread, 1 teaspoon reduced-sugar jam
or marmalade, 1 shredded-wheat biscuit with 1/2
cup milk, 1/2 cup unsweetened orange, grapefruit, or
pineapple juice.

Light meal
Either 1 Pizza Toast (see recipe, page 262) or 1 Lean Cuisine French Bread Pizza, any variety, side salad with oil-free dressing;
or 1½ ounces Cheddar cheese or 3 ounces reduced-fat Cheddar-style cheese, 3-inch piece French bread or 1 large slice bread, mustard, lettuce.

Main meal
Family Choice: 1 portion Chicken Curry (see recipe, page 275), ½ cup rice, 2 teaspoons chutney.
Quick and Easy: 2 chicken tacos made with 2 taco shells, 3 ounces shredded chicken or turkey, 1 chopped tomato, 3 tablespoons taco sauce, ½ cup refried beans.
Heat and Serve: 3 El Charrito Chicken Enchiladas.
Takeout: 2 regular tacos.

Day 7

Breakfast
Either 2 medium poached eggs, 2 slices bread, 2 teaspoons reduced-sugar jelly, ½ cup unsweetened orange, grapefruit, or pineapple juice;
or 2 slices crisply cooked lean bacon or ham, 1 slice whole-wheat toast, ½ cup milk, ¼ cantaloupe.

Light meal
Either 1 10½-ounce can cream of tomato soup prepared with water, 1 small roll, 1 small apple;
or 1 3½-ounce can salmon or sardines or tuna, well drained, 1 small roll or slice bread, side salad with oil-free dressing.

Main meal

Family Choice: 4 ounces lean roast beef, leg of lamb or pork, 1 small baked potato, 1/2 cup spinach or broccoli, 1/3 cup peas, 2 teaspoons mint, horseradish or apple sauce, 1 small pear.

Quick and Easy: 1 Swanson Gravy and Sliced Meat Entree, 1/2 cup peas and carrots, 1/3 cup instant mashed potatoes.

Heat and Serve: 1 Le Menu Yankee Pot Roast, 1 small banana.

Takeout: Same as Day 4.

Sunday brunch exchange

If you prefer, have the following brunch instead of both the Day 7 breakfast and the light meal (so you have just a brunch and main meal today): 1/2 cantaloupe or 1/4 honeydew or 1 cup orange juice, 1 medium egg, dry-fried, 2 breakfast sausage links, well fried or grilled, 1 potato pancake, dry-fried, 1 slice bacon, well grilled; 1 medium slice bread with 1 teaspoon diet margarine.

Day 8

Breakfast

Same as Day 1.

Light meal

Either 3 ounces leftover lean roast meat or lean boiled ham, 1 medium slice bread with a little mustard, 1 sliced tomato, lettuce leaves;
or 1 3-ounce hamburger, broiled, on 1 medium slice toast, 1 sliced tomato, mustard or ketchup.

Main meal

Family Choice: 1 serving Fettuccine with Ham (see recipe, page 279), side salad with oil-free dressing.

Quick and Easy: 4-ounce ham steak, 2 ounces oven fries or 1 small baked potato, 1/4 cup peas.

Heat and Serve: **Either** 1 Armour Ham Steak Dinner;

or 1 Budget Gourmet Pasta Shells with Beef, both with side salad with oil-free dressing, 1 apple.

Takeout: Arby's Beef 'n Cheddar Sandwich or Hot Ham 'n Cheese Sandwich.

Day 9

Breakfast

Same as Day 2.

Light meal

Either 5-inch cheese-and-tomato pizza, side salad with oil-free dressing;

or same as Day 6.

Main meal

Family Choice: 1 serving Turkey Meat Loaf (see recipe, page 273), 1/4 cup instant mashed potatoes, 1/2 cup green beans;

or 1 portion Chili Con Carne (see recipe, page 285), 1/4 cup boiled rice, side salad with oil-free dressing.

Quick and Easy: **Either** 4-ounce lean steak, broiled, 1/4 cup instant mashed potatoes, 1/2 cup green beans;

or 1 cup Van de Kamp's Chili with Beans, 1/4 cup boiled rice, side salad with oil-free dressing.

Heat and Serve: 1 Patio Cheese Enchilada Dinner.

Takeout: **Either** 1 Wendy's Taco Salad;
or 1 Taco Bell Beef Burrito.

Day 10

Breakfast
Same as Day 3.

Light meal
Either 1 medium egg, dry-fried or poached, 3
ounces oven fries, 1 tomato;
or 1 egg, hard-cooked, 2 slices bread with lettuce, 2
teaspoons reduced-calorie mayonnaise.

Main meal
Family Choice: 1 serving Sweet-and-Sour Pork (see
recipe, page 290), 1/4 cup boiled rice or boiled noodles, 1/2 cup chilled broccoli with oil-free dressing.
Quick and Easy: 1 average trimmed pork chop,
broiled, 1 medium boiled potato, 1/4 cup peas, 1 portion Barbecue Sauce (see recipe, page 261) or 2 tablespoons stuffing made from package mix.
Heat and Serve: 1 cup La Choy Sweet and Sour
Pork, with 1 banana, side salad with oil-free dressing.
Takeout: 1 McDonald's Chicken McNuggets, regular
size, with sweet-and-sour sauce.

Day 11

Breakfast
Same as Day 4.

Light meal
Either 3 fish sticks, baked, 1/4 cup instant mashed potatoes, 1/4 cup peas or carrots;
or 1 3 1/2-ounce can tuna, sardines, or salmon, well drained, 1 medium slice bread with 2 teaspoons reduced-calorie mayonnaise, 1 tomato.

Main meal
Family Choice: 1 frankfurter, 1/2 cup baked beans, 3 ounces oven fries.
Quick and Easy: Same as Family Choice.
Heat and Serve: 1 Armour Salisbury Steak Dinner.
Takeout: Dairy Queen DQ Hounder.

Day 12

Breakfast
Same as Day 5.

Light meal
Either cheese toast: 2 slices bread topped with 1 portion Cheese Sauce (see recipe, page 259), 1 sliced tomato over top and browned under broiler;
or 1 1/2 ounces Cheddar cheese or 2 ounces Edam or Brie with 5 saltines or 3 crispbreads, 1 apple.

Main meal
Family Choice: 1 portion Tuna Florentine (see recipe, page 266), 1 medium boiled potato, side salad with oil-free dressing.

Quick and Easy: 2 fish cakes, or 1 crispy-battered cod steak, 3 ounces oven fries, 1/4 cup peas or corn.
Heat and Serve: 1 Stouffer's Scallop and Shrimp Mariner.
Takeout: **Either** 1 McDonald's Filet-O-Fish;
or 1 Burger King Whaler Sandwich.

Day 13

Breakfast
Same as Day 6.

Light meal
Either 4-ounce beefburger, broiled; 3 ounces oven fries, ketchup or mustard;
or 4 ounces very lean ham, 1 average bread roll with lettuce and tomato, 1 teaspoon reduced-calorie mayonnaise.

Main meal
Family Choice: **Either** 1 portion Moussaka (see recipe, page 285), side salad with oil-free dressing;
or 1 portion Beef Enchiladas (see recipe, page 286).
Quick and Easy: 3 Mexican taco shells, filled with 1/2 can beef taco filling, topped with taco sauce, chopped lettuce, and tomato.
Heat and Serve: 1 Banquet International Mexican-Style Dinner.
Takeout: **Either** 1 Taco Bell Beef Burrito;
or 1 McDonald's Quarterpounder, without cheese.

Day 14

Breakfast
Same as Day 7.

Light meal
Either Stouffer's Lean Cuisine French Bread Pizza, any variety, side salad with oil-free dressing; **or** 2 ounces corned beef spread, 3 crispbreads or 1 slice bread, lettuce, tomato, 1 apple.

Main meal
Family Choice: 4 ounces roast chicken or turkey, skin removed, 1 small baked potato, 1/2 cup mixed peas and carrots, 2 tablespoons packaged stuffing.
Quick and Easy: 1 roast chicken breast, skin removed, 1/2 cup instant mashed potatoes or 1 small baked potato or 2 thin slices bread, 1/4 cup peas or corn, salad with oil-free dressing.
Heat and Serve: 1 Stouffer's Cashew Chicken in Sauce with Rice, side salad with oil-free dressing;
Takeout: **Either** 1 Hardee's Turkey Club Sandwich; **or** 1 Church's Fried Chicken Breast with 2 Hush Puppies.

Sunday brunch exchange
Same as Day 7.

DIET THREE

(approximately 1,500 calories a day)

Every day:
  You may have Unlimiteds from the list on page 108.

You should have your two Snacks—your milk or yogurt, and your fruit.

You can pick Treats/Extras up to 250 calories a day from the lists on pages 197–202.

Day 1

Breakfast
Either 2 slices bread with 2 teaspoons reduced-sugar jam or marmalade, 1 diet fruit yogurt, 1/2 cup unsweetened orange, grapefruit, or pineapple juice; **or** 11/2 ounces breakfast cereal of choice with 1 cup milk and 1 teaspoon sugar, 1/2 cup unsweetened orange, grapefruit, or pineapple juice.

Light meal
Either 3 ounces sliced turkey breast, 1/4 cup corn, 1 slice bread with 1 teaspoon reduced-calorie mayonnaise; **or** 1 medium cooked chicken breast, skin removed, 1 salad or 1 slice bread.

Main meal
Family Choice: 1 serving Marinated Ginger Pork (see recipe, page 292), 1/4 cup peas, 1 small baked sweet potato or 1 white potato.
Quick and Easy: 1 frankfurter, 1/2 cup baked beans, 1 diet yogurt or small apple.
Heat and Serve: 1 average Beef Pot Pie.
Takeout: 1 Wendy's Hot Stuffed Baked Potato with Chili and Cheese.

Day 2

Breakfast
Either 2 slices bread with 4 teaspoons reduced-sugar jam or marmalade, 1/2 grapefruit or 1/2 cup canned grapefruit sections;
or 2 shredded-wheat biscuits, 1 cup milk, 1/2 grapefruit or 1/2 canned grapefruit sections.

Light meal
Either 2 ounces Cheddar cheese, melted on 2 slices toast, topped with 1 sliced tomato;
or 2 ounces Cheddar cheese with slice bread, 5 Saltines, 1 apple.

Main meal
Family Choice: 1 serving Beef Enchiladas (see recipe, page 286), 1/2 cup corn, 1/2 cup green beans.
Quick and Easy: 1 Stouffer's Chili Con Carne with Beans, 1/2 cup rice, 5 saltines.
Heat and Serve: 1 Patio Beef Enchilada Dinner.
Takeout: 1 Taco Bell Double Beef Supreme Burrito.

Day 3

Breakfast
Either 3 slices crisp bacon, 1 slice bread with 1/2 cup unsweetened orange, grapefruit, or pineapple juice;
or 2 medium slices bread with 2 teaspoons reduced-sugar jam or marmalade, 1 banana or diet yogurt.

Light meal
Either 1 10.75-ounce can ready-to-serve Campbell's Chunky Chicken Soup, 1 slice bread, 1 apple;
or 3 ounces very lean ham, 1 slice bread, 2 crisp-

breads, tomato salad with reduced-calorie Italian
dressing.

Main meal

Family Choice: 1 serving Potato Frittata (see recipe,
page 265), 1/2 cup peas, 1 cup stewed tomatoes, 1
small roll.
Quick and Easy: 2 medium eggs, dry-fried, 3 ounces
oven fries, 1/4 cup peas, 1 slice bread.
Heat and Serve: 1 Mrs. Smith's Mushroom Quiche.
Takeout: 3 slices Pizza Hut Thin-n Crispy Pizza Supreme.

Day 4

Breakfast

Same as Day 2.

Light meal

Either 1 3-ounce beefburger, broiled, on roll;
or 1 3 1/2-ounce can tuna, well drained, 1 small roll,
1 tablespoon reduced-calorie mayonnaise, lettuce,
and tomato.

Main meal

Family Choice: 1 portion Spring Vegetable Lasagna
Rolls (see recipe, page 282), 1 slice bread, large salad
with oil-free dressing.
Quick and Easy: 4-ounce beefburger, well grilled or
deep-fried, 3 ounces oven fries, 1/2 cup corn, 1 orange.
Heat and Serve: **Either** 1 Stouffer's Lasagna;
or Green Giant Lasagna with Meat Sauce.
Takeout: 1 regular hamburger and regular french
fries.

Day 5

Breakfast
Same as Day 1.

Light meal
Either 2 medium eggs, poached or scrambled on 1 slice toast, 1 diet yogurt;

or 1 egg, hard-cooked, with large salad, 1 teaspoon reduced-calorie mayonnaise, 1 small pita pocket, 1 diet yogurt.

Main meal
Family Choice: 1 portion Fish Kebabs (see recipe, page 270), 1/2 cup boiled rice, large salad with oil-free dressing.

Quick and Easy: 4 fish sticks, baked, 1/2 cup instant mashed potatoes or 3 ounces oven fries, 1/4 cup peas, 1 banana.

Heat and Serve: 1 Gorton's Seafood Lover's Fillet Almondine, 1/2 cup broccoli, 1/2 cup stewed tomatoes.

Takeout: 1 Burger King Whaler Sandwich.

Day 6

Breakfast
Either 3 slices crisp bacon, 1 slice toast, diet margarine, 1/2 cup unsweetened orange, grapefruit, or pineapple juice;

or 2 shredded-wheat biscuits with 1/2 cup milk, 1 slice toast with 2 teaspoons reduced-sugar jam or marmalade.

Light meal

Either 1 Pizza Toast (see recipe, page 262);
or 1 Lean Cuisine French Bread Pizza, any variety;
or 1 1/2 ounces Cheddar cheese or 3 ounces reduced-fat Cheddar-style cheese, 3 inches French bread or 1 large slice bread with 1 pear.

Main meal

Family Choice: 1 serving Chicken Curry (see recipe, page 275), 1/2 cup boiled rice, 1/4 cup plain non-fat yogurt with chopped cucumber.
Quick and Easy: 3 ounces Tyson Chicken Patties, 1/2 cup mashed potatoes, 1/2 cup peas, 1 banana.
Heat and Serve: Stouffer's Cashew Chicken in Sauce, with rice.
Takeout: Kentucky Fried Chicken Side Breast with Corn on the Cob and Mashed Potatoes.

Day 7

Breakfast

Either 2 slices crisp bacon, 1 medium egg, poached, 1 slice toast;
or 3 ounces cooked lean ham, 2 slices toast;
or same as Day 1.

Light meal

Either 1 10 1/2-ounce can Campbell's Cream of Tomato Soup prepared with water, 1 small roll, 1 apple;
or 1 3 1/2-ounce can salmon or sardines or tuna, well drained, 1 small roll or 1 slice bread, side salad with oil-free dressing.

Main meal

Family Choice: 4 ounces lean roast beef or leg of lamb or pork; 1 small baked potato, 1/2 cup spinach or broccoli, 1/3 cup peas, 2 teaspoons mint, and horseradish or apple sauce.

Quick and Easy: 1 Swanson Gravy and Sliced Meat Entree, 1/2 cup instant mashed potatoes, 1/2 cup peas, 1 diet yogurt.

Heat and Serve: 1 Beef Pot Pie.

Takeout: Same as Day 4.

Sunday brunch exchange

If you prefer, have the following brunch instead of both the Day 7 breakfast and the light meal (so you just have a brunch and main meal today): 1/2 cantaloupe or 1/4 honeydew, 1 cup orange juice, 2 eggs, dry-fried, 1 breakfast sausage, well fried or grilled, 1 potato pancake, dry-fried or grilled, 2 slices bacon, well grilled, 1 slice bread with 1 teaspoon diet margarine.

Day 8

Breakfast

Same as Day 1.

Light meal

Either 3-ounce beefburger, broiled, 1/4 cup instant mashed potatoes, 4 tablespoons peas, 1 diet yogurt; **or** 3 ounces leftover roast meat, lean only, 1 slice bread or 2 thin slices bread with a little mustard, sliced tomato, lettuce leaves.

Main meal
Family Choice: 1 serving Fettuccine with Ham (see recipe, page 279), salad with oil-free dressing, 1 small orange or apple.
Quick and Easy: 5-ounce ham steak, 4 ounces oven fries or 1 small baked potato, 1/2 cup peas or lima beans.
Heat and Serve: **Either** 1 Armour Ham Steak Dinner, side salad with oil-free dressing;
or 1 Budget Gourmet Pasta Shells with Beef, side salad with oil-free dressing, 1 orange or apple, plus extra 100 calories' worth of any Extra (see pages 197–202).
Takeout: Arby's Beef 'n Cheddar or Super Roast Beef Sandwich.

Day 9

Breakfast
Same as Day 2.

Light meal
Either 5-inch cheese-and-tomato pizza, side salad with oil-free dressing;
or same as Day 6.

Main meal
Family Choice: **Either** 1 serving Turkey Meat Loaf (see recipe, page 273), 1/2 cup mashed potatoes or 1 medium baked potato, 1/2 cup green beans;
or 1 portion Chili Con Carne (see recipe, page 285), 1/2 cup boiled rice, side salad with oil-free dressing.
Quick and Easy: **Either** 4 ounces lean steak, broiled or grilled, 4 ounces oven fries, 1/4 cup peas or corn;

or 1 can Armour Chili with Beans, side salad with oil-free dressing, 1 apple.

Heat and Serve: 1 Patio Cheese Enchilada Dinner, 1 banana.

Takeout: 1 Wendy's Hot Stuffed Baked Potato with Chili and Cheese.

Day 10

Breakfast
Same as Day 3.

Light meal
Either 1 medium egg, dry-fried or poached, 4 ounces oven fries, 1 tomato;
or 1 medium egg, hard-cooked, 2 slices bread with lettuce, 2 teaspoons reduced-calorie mayonnaise.

Main meal
Family Choice: 1 serving Sweet-and-Sour Pork (see recipe, page 290), 1/2 boiled rice or boiled noodles, 1/2 cup broccoli, large salad with reduced-calorie dressing.

Quick and Easy: 1 average trimmed pork chop, broiled, 1 medium boiled potato, 1/4 cup peas or broccoli, 1 portion Barbecue Sauce (see recipe, page 261) or 2 tablespoons stuffing from package.

Heat and Serve: 1 La Choy Sweet and Sour Pork Dinner with large salad with oil-free dressing, 1 orange.

Day 11

Breakfast
Same as Day 4.

Light meal
Either 3 fish sticks, baked, 3 tablespoons instant mashed potatoes, 4 tablespoons peas or carrots;
or 1 3 1/2-ounce can tuna or sardines or salmon, well drained, 1 medium slice bread with 2 teaspoons reduced-calorie mayonnaise.

Main meal
Family Choice: 1 frankfurter, 1/2 cup baked beans, 5 ounces oven fries.
Quick and Easy: Same as Family Choice.
Heat and Serve: 1 Armour Salisbury Steak Dinner, 1 small apple.
Takeout: 3 slices Pizza Hut Thin-n Crispy Pizza Supreme.

Day 12

Breakfast
Same as Day 5.

Light meal
Either cheese toast—2 slices toast topped with 1 portion Cheese Sauce (see recipe, page 259), with 1 sliced tomato on top, and browned under broiler;
or 1 1/2 ounces Cheddar cheese or 2 ounces Edam or Brie with 5 saltines or 3 crispbreads, 1 apple.

Main meal

Family Choice: 1 portion Tuna Florentine (see recipe, page 266), 1 medium boiled potato, 1 cup broccoli, 1 apple.

Quick and Easy: 2 fish cakes, dry-fried, or 1 crispy-battered cod steak, 3 ounces oven fries, 1/2 cup peas or corn, 1 diet yogurt.

Heat and Serve: Stouffer's Scallop and Shrimp Mariner, 1/2 cup green beans.

Takeout: 1 McDonald's Filet-O-Fish Sandwich, side salad with diet dressing.

Day 13

Breakfast

Same as Day 6.

Light meal

Either 4-ounce broiled beefburger, 3 ounces oven fries, ketchup or mustard, lettuce, tomato;

or 4 ounces very lean ham, 1 average roll with 1 teaspoon reduced-calorie mayonnaise, lettuce, tomato.

Main meal

Family Choice: **Either** 1 portion Moussaka (see recipe, page 285);

or 1 portion Beef Enchiladas (see recipe, page 286), both with salad, 1 banana or 1 yogurt.

Quick and Easy: 3 Mexican taco shells filled with 1/2 can beef taco filling, topped with taco sauce and chopped salad items of choice, salad, banana.

Heat and Serve: 1 Patio Beef Enchilada Dinner.

Takeout: Same as Day 3 or 4.

Day 14

Breakfast
Same as Day 7.

Light meal
Either 1 Stouffer's Lean Cuisine French Bread Pizza, any variety, salad;
or 2 ounces corned beef spread, 3 crispbreads or 1 slice bread, lettuce, tomato.

Main meal
Family Choice: 4 ounces roast chicken or turkey, skin removed, 1 medium baked potato, 1/2 cup mixed peas and carrots, 4 tablespoons packaged stuffing.
Quick and Easy: 1 large roast chicken breast, skin removed, 1/2 cup instant mashed potatoes or 2 medium slices bread, 1/4 cup peas or corn, salad with oil-free dressing.
Heat and Serve: 1 Swanson's Chicken Nuggets Platter, side salad with oil-free dressing.
Takeout: 1 portion McDonald's Chicken McNuggets (6) with regular french fries.

Sunday brunch exchange
Same as Day 7.

✤ 8. ✤

The Junk Food Diet—3

THE PICK-YOUR-OWN PLAN

Now you're ready to pick your own junk food diet—and it's simplicity itself, with the help of the meal listings that follow. All you have to do is pick meals and extras to reach your own dieting calorie level—1,000, 1,250, or 1,500.

To help you, here is a breakdown of the calorie-counted meal categories available for you to choose from. The detailed contents of these categories are given on pages 153–202.

The only things to remember—apart from the rules listed in Chapter 6, which still apply here—are:

- Have no more than one meal from any one meal section a day, and get as much variety into your daily diet as you can. For instance, if you had an egg meal for breakfast, don't have eggs for lunch and dinner as well.
- Some vegetables are included within many meals. You should also use the vegetables on the Unlimiteds list as much as you like, and if you want extra vegetables, there are plenty to choose from within the listings.

Pick Your Own Reference Guide

Meals	Calorie Levels
Breakfasts and Snacks, cold	200, 250, 300
Breakfasts and Snacks, hot	300
Light Meals, cold	250, 300, 400
Light Meals, Brunches, and Suppers, hot	300, 400, 500
Toast Meals	250, 300, 400
Bread and Sandwich Meals	250, 300, 400
Potato Meals	250, 400
Main Meals, Family Choice	300, 400, 500, 600
Main Meals, Quick and Easy	300, 400, 500, 600
Main Meals, Heat and Serve	300, 400, 500, 600
Top Takeouts	300, 400, 500, 600, 700
Vegetables, Pasta, and Rice	25, 50, 75, 100, 150
Fruits and Juices	25, 50, 100
Milk and Yogurt	50, 100
Treats, Snacks, and Extras	25, 50, 75, 100, 150, 200, 250

- Try to get a daily portion of milk or yogurt and fruit, as you did on the Set Diet.
- Your daily maximum Treats/Extras allowance is still 100 calories if you're on 1,000 calories a day,

150 calories if you're on 1,250 calories a day, and 250 if you're on 1,500 calories a day. Select them from the lists on pages 197 to 202. But if you prefer not to use these calories on Treats, you can, of course, use them on other foods listed.

• Try to have several meals/snacks a day rather than just one big meal. If you're on 1,000 calories a day, the maximum calorie count for any one meal should be 500. If you're on 1,250 or 1,500, the maximum should be 600. The only exception to this rule is that if you're on 1,250 or 1,500 calories, you can have an occasional Takeout of 700. But on those "high takeout" days, you would be wise to forgo your day's Treats allowance and spend the calories on something else, such as a fruit and yogurt snack or a small meal.

Don't forget, you can return to the Set Diet any time you like, and you should move down a calorie band if your weight loss slows right down or stops.

As to brand names, when I haven't specified one before a product, any brand will do: For instance, fish sticks, fish cakes, and instant mashed potatoes vary by hardly any calories from brand to brand. But sometimes calories do vary widely, so when I've specified a brand name it's best to stick to it, which is why I've used only widely available brands or top supermarket labels.

Before you start, take a good look through the listings to familiarize yourself with them. Spend some time planning out some combinations that appeal to you and working out meal patterns that are compatible with the way you live.

Examples

Following are two examples of how you might plan out a day's menu from the lists, according to your own needs.

. Tina is on 1,250 calories a day. She is at work and needs a quick breakfast, a packed lunch, and a very quick family evening meal during the week. She chooses:

    Cold Breakfast—200 calories
    Cold Lunch—300 calories
    Fruit—50 calories
    Quick and Easy Main Meal—400 calories
    Dessert from Treats list—100 calories
    Extra butter from Extras list—100 calories
    Milk for use in drinks—100 calories

However, on a Sunday she prefers a late-morning brunch, and a main meal with dessert in the evening, so she chooses:

    Brunch—400 calories
    Sandwich Meal—250 calories
    Main Meal—300 calories
    Dessert (from Treats list)—200 calories
    Fruit—50 calories
    Milk—50 calories

Emily, a teen-ager on 1,500 calories, likes to snack during the day, and this Saturday she wants to look forward to a takeout supper with her friends. This is what she chooses:

    Cold Breakfast—200 calories
    Early lunch of a sandwich meal—250 calories

Fruit—50 calories
Snack of a toast meal—250 calories
Diet yogurt—50 calories
Takeout dinner—700 calories

She prefers not to use her remaining calories as a Treats allowance, having her takeout meal and a breakfast instead.

Plan out your own meals this way, and you'll find losing weight to be a pleasure.

PLEASE NOTE: When using the listings that follow, you should pick one item from the first column and then stay within that horizontal ruled section when picking the rest of your meal from columns two and/or three.

Cold Breakfasts and Snacks—200 calories

Pick one of these	*Plus*	
2 shredded-wheat biscuits 1 cup Cheerios	1 cup skim milk	

Pick one of these	*Plus*	*Plus one of these*
1 cup cornflakes ¾ cup frosted flakes ¾ cup Post Fruit & Fibre ½ cup raisin bran	½ cup skim milk	Any 1 portion from 50-calorie fruit selection on page 196 ½ cup unsweetened orange or

Pick one of these	Plus	Plus one of these
1 cup Kellogg's Special K 1 cup Kellogg's Total 1 cup Kellogg's Wheaties		grapefruit juice
1/2 cup Kellogg's All Bran 1/2 cup Kellogg's Bran Buds 3/4 cup bran flakes	1/2 cup skim milk	1/2 banana 1 thin slice bread, plain
1 8-ounce non-fat plain yogurt	1 banana 1/2 grapefruit with 1 teaspoon honey	
1 slice bread	3 teaspoons honey 3 teaspoons marmalade 3 teaspoons jam 6 teaspoons reduced-sugar jam 1 ounce low-fat cream cheese	Any 1 portion from 50-calorie fruit selection on page 196
1 plain bagel		

Pick one of these	Plus	Plus one of these
2 slices bread 1 English muffin 1/2 plain bagel	3 teaspoons jam 3 teaspoons marmalade 6 teaspoons reduced-sugar jam 6 teaspoons reduced-sugar marmalade 1 portion from 50-calorie fruit selection on page 196	

Cold Breakfasts and Snacks—250 calories

Pick one of these	Plus	Plus one of these
1 8-ounce container non-fat plain yogurt 1/2 cup Kellogg's Müeslix	1/2 banana 1/2 cup skim milk	1 thin slice toast Any 1 portion from 50-calorie fruit selection on page 196

| 1 cup cornflakes
3/4 cup frosted flakes
3/4 cup Kellogg's Fruit & Fibre
1/2 cup raisin bran
1 cup Kellogg's Special K | 1/2 cup skim milk | 1 slice bread from a thin-cut loaf with 1 teaspoon jam or marmalade or jelly |

Pick one of these	Plus	Plus one of these
1 cup Kellogg's Total		
1 cup Kellogg's Wheaties		
1 average bread roll	1 ounce Cheddar cheese	
2 thin slices bread	1 non-fat plain yogurt	
	6 teaspoons reduced-sugar jam	
	6 teaspoons reduced-sugar marmalade	
	2 tablespoons cream cheese	
2 thin slices bread	1 banana	
	2 ounces lean ham	
	1 8-ounce container low-fat plain yogurt	

Cold Breakfasts and Snacks—300 calories

Pick one of these	Plus	Plus one of these
1 cup cornflakes	1/2 cup skim milk	1 slice bread with reduced-sugar jam plus
3/4 cup frosted flakes		

Pick one of these	Plus	Plus one of these
3/4 cup Kellogg's Fruit & Fibre 1/2 cup raisin bran 1 cup Kellogg's Special K 1 cup Kellogg's Total 1 cup Kellogg's Wheaties		1/2 cup unsweetened orange or grapefruit juice or 1 cup tomato juice
2 shredded-wheat biscuits	1/2 cup skim milk 4 ounces semi-skim milk	1 banana 1 slice bread with 1 teaspoon jam or marmalade
2 slices bread	1 ounce Cheddar cheese 3 slices lean ham 2 slices bacon, crisp, well drained 2 breakfast sausage links, well drained	
1 serving instant oatmeal	3/4 cup skim milk	
2 medium eggs, dry-fried	1 slice bacon, crisp, well drained	1 thin slice bread

Pick one of these	Plus	Plus one of these
1 medium egg, dry-fried	2 slices bacon, crisp, well drained	1 crispbread 1/2 grapefruit

---

Breakfasts and Snacks, hot—300 calories

Pick one of these	Plus	Plus one of these
1 medium egg, dry fried 2 medium eggs, poached	1 slice bacon, crisp, well drained 2 breakfast sausage links, well grilled and drained	1 slice toast 2 slices Melba toast or rye crispbread

---

Light Meals, cold—250 calories

Pick one of these	Plus	Plus one of these
1 hot dog 3 ounces very lean ham 3 ounces chicken meat or chicken roll 1 ounce corned beef 1 ounce Cheddar cheese 2 ounces reduced-fat Cheddar cheese 1 ounce Edam, Brie, or Dan-	1 small potato, boiled 1 slice bread 3 crispbreads 5 saltines 1 small pita pocket 1/4 cup potato or macaroni salad	1 teaspoon mayonnaise 2 teaspoons reduced-calorie mayonnaise 2 teaspoons diet margarine

Pick one of these	*Plus*	*Plus one of these*
ish blue cheese		
1 egg, hard-cooked		
1 3 1/2-ounce can pink salmon, well drained		
1 3 1/2-ounce can water-packed tuna, well drained		
3 ounces lean roast beef		
2 ounces cold cuts, such as bologna, salami		

Light Meals, cold—300 calories

Pick one of these	*Plus*	*Plus one of these*
2 medium eggs, hard-cooked	2-inch slice French bread	
1 large cold cooked chicken breast, skin removed	2 thin slices bread from small loaf	
	3 ounces corn salad	
1/3 cup hummus	1 pita pocket	
2 ounces corned beef	3 crispbreads	
	1 slice bread	
1 1/2 ounces Cheddar cheese	1/2 cup potato salad, macaroni salad, or coleslaw	
1 1/2 ounces Danish blue		
1 3 1/2-ounce can	1/3 cup three-bean salad	

Pick one of these	Plus	Plus one of these
salmon, well drained		
1 3½-ounce can sardines, well drained		

Light Meals, cold—400 calories

Pick one of these	Plus	Plus one of these
2 ounces Cheddar cheese	4-inch slice French bread	1 tomato 2 teaspoons diet margarine
3 ounces reduced-fat Cheddar-style cheese	4-inch slice French bread	2 teaspoons diet margarine
¾ cup tuna salad	1 small pita pocket	chopped salad 1 tablespoon reduced-calorie mayonnaise
1 serving Paradise Chicken (see recipe, page 277)	¼ cup cold cooked rice tossed with oil-free dressing ½ mini pita pocket 1 thin slice bread	

Light Meals, Brunches, and Suppers, hot—300 calories

Pick one of these	*Plus*	*Plus one of these*
3 fish sticks, baked	1 small potato, boiled	Any 1 portion from 50-calorie fruit selection on page 196
1 fish cake, baked	1/4 cup rice, boiled	
1 5-ounce fish fillet, breaded	1 slice bread	
1 small chicken breast, skin removed	2 ounces oven fries	3 tablespoons sweet corn
3 breakfast sausage links, well drained	1 egg, dry-fried	1/2 cup peas
3-ounce ham steak		1/4 cup baked beans
2 1/2-ounce Banquet Hot Bites, Breast Tenders		

1 medium egg, dry-fried	2 ounces oven fries

Chicken and Broccoli Casserole (see recipe, page 274)	1/4 cup instant mashed potatoes
1 portion Spanish Scramble (see recipe, page 264)	1 slice bread

Pick one of these	Plus	Plus one of these
1½ cups any of these soups: cream of celery chicken mushroom minestrone vegetable lentil pea and ham	1 average roll 2-inch slice French bread	Any 1 portion from 50-calorie fruit selection on page 196 1 tablespoon diet margarine

Stouffer's Escalloped Chicken and Noodles Any Stouffer's Lean Cuisine	side salad with oil-free dressing	

Stouffer's Beef and Spinach Stuffed Pasta Shells with Tomato Sauce Stouffer's Beef Stew Stouffer's Ham and Swiss Cheese Crepes with Cheese Sauce		

Light Meals, Brunches, and Suppers, hot—400 calories

Pick one of these	Plus	Plus one of these
1 serving Fish Kebabs (see	2 ounces oven fries	

Pick one of these	Plus	Plus one of these
recipe, page 270) 1 serving Beef Goulash (see recipe, page 287) 1 serving Vegetable Lasagna Rolls (see recipe, page 282)	1 slice bread 1 small potato, boiled	
Le Menu Chopped Sirloin Beef Le Menu Beef Sirloin Tips Budget Gourmet Chicken with Fettuccine Banquet Fried Chicken Dinner Armour Veal Parmigiana		
1 medium egg, dry-fried	2 breakfast sausage links, well grilled and drained	4 ounces oven fries
1 4-ounce beefburger, broiled or baked	1 burger roll	lettuce and tomatoes

Pick one of these	*Plus*	*Plus one of these*
2 medium eggs, dry-fried 4 fish sticks, baked	4 ounces oven fries	
1 serving Tandoori Chicken (see recipe, page 272)	3/4 cup rice, boiled, plus 1/2 cup peas 1 pita pocket, plus 1 table-spoon chut-ney, plus 1/2 cup plain non-fat yogurt	
1 portion Ri-sotto (see rec-ipe, page 283) 1 portion Chicken Curry (see recipe, page 275)	Any 1 serving from 50-calo-rie fruit selec-tion on page 196 green beans and broccoli	1 tablespoon grated Parme-san cheese 1/2 cup green peas 1 cup broccoli or green beans
1 portion Chili Con Carne (see recipe, page 285)	1/3 cup boiled rice	
1 Tuna Pita (see recipe, page 263)		

Brunches—500 calories

Choose one of the following brunches:

1 medium egg, dry-fried
1 slice lean, crisp bacon, well-drained
2 breakfast sausage links, well grilled and drained
1 potato pancake or hash browns, dry-fried or baked
1 slice bread or 1 extra egg
1 teaspoon diet margarine
1/2 cup unsweetened orange or grapefruit juice

1/4 cantaloupe or 1/8 honeydew
1 waffle
2 slices lean, crisp bacon, well grilled and drained
2 tablespoons syrup
1 teaspoon diet margarine

1/2 grapefruit or 1 large orange, sectioned
1/2 cup cooked sliced potato, sautéed and drained
2 medium eggs, dry-fried
2 slices lean, crisp bacon, well grilled and drained

---

2 breakfast sausage links, well grilled and drained
2 medium eggs, poached
2 slices toast
1 teaspoon diet margarine

Toast Meals—250 calories

Pick one of these

2 medium eggs, poached
1 ounce Cheddar cheese
and 1 sliced tomato
2 ounces lean ham, plus
1 teaspoon mustard
and 1 teaspoon honey

Plus one of these

1 slice bread, toasted,
with 2 teaspoons diet
margarine
3 inches French bread,
split and toasted
1/2 English muffin

Pick one of these

- 1 ounce turkey, plus 1
  ounce low-fat Swiss
  cheese
- 2 ounces reduced-fat
  Cheddar cheese, melted

Plus one of these

- 1/2 plain bagel
- 1 small pita pocket

Toast Meals—300 calories

Pick one of these

- 2 medium eggs, scram-
  bled with 1/4 cup milk
  and 2 teaspoons low-fat
  spread
- 2 ounces Cheshire or
  Edam cheese, melted
- 1/2 cup chicken à la king
- 2 ounces low-fat moz-
  zarella cheese, shred-
  ded, plus 1 tomato,
  sliced
- 1 cup mushrooms, sliced,
  stir-fried in 1 table-
  spoon butter
- 1 3 1/2-ounce can sardines
  in oil, well drained
- 1 serving Spanish Scramble (see recipe, page
  264)

Plus one of these

- 1 slice bread, toasted,
  with 2 teaspoons diet
  margarine
- 3 inches French bread,
  split and toasted
- 1/2 English muffin
- 1/2 plain bagel
- 1 small pita pocket

---

1 Pizza Toast (see recipe, page 262)

Toast Meals—400 calories

Pick one of these

- 1 8-ounce can Heinz
  baked beans with pork

Plus one of these

- 1 slice bread, toasted

Pick one of these   *Plus one of these*

sausages or burger
bites
1 4¹/₂-ounce can sardines
in tomato or mustard
sauce
¹/₃ Stouffer's Welsh Rare-
bit
¹/₂ Stouffer's Lobster
Newburg
¹/₂ Stouffer's Creamed
Chipped Beef

Bread and Sandwich Meals—250 calories

Pick one of these   *Plus one of these*

1 medium egg, hard-   2 thin slices bread
cooked, plus 2 tea-
spoons reduced-calorie
mayonnaise
2 ounces very lean ham,
plus 2 teaspoons re-
duced-calorie mayon-
naise or sweet relish
2¹/₂ ounces chicken or
turkey roll
2 ounces lean roast beef
or pork
1 3¹/₂-ounce can shrimp,
drained, plus 2 tea-
spoons reduced-calorie
mayonnaise
1 heaping tablespoon
peanut butter
1 Kraft Single and 1
ounce lean ham
1 ounce Bel Paese cheese
1 ounce Edam cheese
1¹/₂ ounces reduced-fat
Cheddar-style cheese

Bread and Sandwich Meals—300 calories

Pick one of these

1 1/2 ounces Cheddar

2 ounces reduced-fat
Cheddar-style cheese

1 ounce corned beef, plus
1 teaspoon pickle

1 slice bologna, 2 lettuce
leaves, 1 teaspoon mus-
tard

1 3 1/2-ounce can pink
salmon, well drained

2 ounces chicken meat,
plus 1 tablespoon re-
duced-calorie mayon-
naise with 1/2 teaspoon
curry powder (optional)

1 tablespoon peanut but-
ter, plus 1 tablespoon
jelly or jam

Plus one of these

2 thin slices bread

1 average bread roll

---

1 Pizza Toast (see recipe,
page 262)

1 Lean Cuisine French
Bread Pizza, any vari-
ety

1 Weight Watchers
Deluxe Combination
Pizza

Bread and Sandwich Meals—400 calories

Pick one of these

1/4 of any 22-ounce pizza

---

1 Tuna Pita (see recipe,
page 263)

Pick one of these

1 pita pocket filled with
    1/2 of 61/2-ounce can
    salmon, with 2 tea-
    spoons reduced-fat
    mayonnaise

Potato Meals—250 calories

Pick one of these	*Plus*	*Plus one of these*
1/2 cup instant mashed potatoes	1 medium egg, poached	1 teaspoon butter
1/2 cup hash browns	2 ounces medium-fat soft cheese	2 teaspoons diet margarine
1/4 cup au gratin potatoes	1/2 cup Birds Eye Broccoli with Creamy Italian Cheese	
1 medium potato, boiled	1/2 cup Birds Eye Mandarine Style International Vegetables	
1 small potato, baked	11/2 cups Birds Eye Mixed Chinese-Style Vegetables	
	2 slices crisp bacon, well drained and crumbled	

Potato Meals—400 calories

Pick one of these	Plus	Plus one of these
1 medium potato, baked 1/2 large sweet potato, baked	2 ounces grated Cheddar cheese 2 ounces very lean ham, chopped, and 1 large egg, poached 2 ounces mozzarella cheese, plus 2 tablespoons spaghetti sauce 1 cup chili with beans	1/2 cup broccoli 1/2 cup green beans 1 tablespoon grated Parmesan cheese 1 tablespoon bacon bits

Main Meals, Family Choice—300 calories

Pick one of these	Plus	Plus one of these
1 portion Turkey Kebabs (see recipe, page 276) 1 portion Shrimp Provençale (see recipe, page 268) 1 serving Chicken and Broccoli Casserole (see	1/2 small potato, boiled 1 medium potato, baked 1/4 cup instant mashed potatoes 1/4 cup rice, boiled 1/2 cup noodles, boiled 2 ounces oven fries	Vegetables or salad of choice from Unlimiteds list

Pick one of these	Plus	Plus one of these
recipe, page 274) 1 serving Fisherman's Soup (see recipe, page 267) 1 serving Pork Chops with Rosemary (see recipe, page 291) 1 serving Tandoori Chicken (see recipe, page 272) 3 ounces lean roast beef, leg of lamb, or pork 3 ounces roast chicken, skin removed	1/4 cup Spanish rice 1/4 cup Rice-A-Roni 1/3 cup plain pasta 2 tablespoons stuffing mix, packaged	

Main Meals, Family Choice—400 calories

Pick one of these	Plus	Plus one of these
4 ounces roast lamb or beef 1/2 of 1-pound pack or tin chili con carne (not including rice) 1 serving Sweet-and-Sour	1 small potato, baked 1/2 cup rice, boiled 1/2 cup noodles, boiled 1/4 cup instant mashed potatoes	Any vegetable or salad item from Unlimiteds list

Pick one of these	*Plus*	*Plus one of these*
Pork (see recipe, page 290)	2 ounces oven fries	
5 ounces lean ham		
1 Chun King Chunky Walnut Chicken		
1 Banquet Gourmet Entree Green Pepper Steak		
1 cup chili with beef and beans		
1 Tyson Swiss 'n Bacon Chicken Sautee		

1 portion Fisherman's Soup (see recipe, page 267)	1 small potato, boiled	Any vegetable or salad item from Unlimiteds list
1 portion Chili Con Carne (see recipe, page 285)	1 small potato, baked	
	1/2 cup rice, boiled	
1 serving Cod Creole (see recipe, page 269)	1/2 cup noodles, boiled	
	1/2 cup Rice-A-Roni	
1 serving Spanish Scramble (see recipe, page 264)	1/2 cup instant mashed potatoes	
1 serving Turkey Kebabs		

Pick one of these	*Plus*	*Plus one of these*
(see recipe, page 276)		

---

1 serving Beef Goulash (see recipe, page 287)	1/2 small potato, baked	
1 portion Beef Stroganoff (see recipe, page 288)	1/2 small potato, boiled	
1 serving Beef Stir-Fry (see recipe, page 289)	1/4 cup rice, boiled	
1 serving Chicken Curry (see recipe, page 275)	1/4 cup noodles, boiled	
1 serving Fish Kebabs (see recipe, page 270)		

---

1 serving Vegetable Lasagna Rolls (see recipe, page 282)	Any 1 portion from 50-calorie fruit selection on page 196)	
1 serving Risotto (see recipe, page 283)		
1 serving Macaroni and Cheese (see		

Pick one of these	*Plus*	*Plus one of these*

recipe, page
278)
1 serving Para-
dise Chicken
(see recipe,
page 277)

Main Meals, Family Choice—500 calories

Pick one of these	*Plus*	*Plus one of these*

1 portion Sweet-
and-Sour
Pork (see rec-
ipe, page 290)
1 portion Tuna
Florentine
(see recipe,
page 266)
1 Banquet Hot
'n Spicy Fried
Chicken
1 Tyson
Chicken
Jambalaya
1 8-ounce Chef
Boyardee
Meatball
Stew
1 Chun King
Sweet and
Sour Pork
1 serving Beef
Stroganoff
(see recipe,
page 288)
1 serving
Chicken

1 small potato,
baked
1/2 cup rice,
boiled
1/2 cup noodles,
boiled
1/4 cup instant
mashed pota-
toes

Pick one of these	Plus	Plus one of these
Curry (see recipe, page 275)		

Pick one of these	Plus	Plus one of these
1 portion Beef Enchiladas (see recipe, page 286)	Any 1 portion from 50-calorie fruit selection on page 196	
1 portion Moussaka (see recipe, page 285)		
1 portion Fettuccine with Ham (see recipe, page 279)		

Main Meals, Family Choice—600 calories

Pick one of these	Plus	Plus one of these
1 serving Moussaka (see recipe, page 285)	1/2 potato, boiled	1/2 cup lima beans
1 serving Beef Enchiladas (see recipe, page 286)	2 ounces oven fries	1/2 cup peas
1 Tyson Chicken Fiesta	1/2 potato, baked	1/2 cup sweet corn
1 Tyson Chicken Parmigiana	1/4 cup rice, boiled	
1 Tyson Sweet and Sour Chicken		

Pick one of these	Plus	Plus one of these
1 Swanson Turkey Pie		
1 Van de Kamp's Sirloin Burrito Grande		

Pick one of these	Plus	Plus one of these
1 serving Pasta Shells with Tuna (see recipe, page 280)	1 large salad with reduced-calorie dressing	
1 serving Spaghetti with Meat Sauce (see recipe, page 281)		
1 Van de Kamp's Chicken Suiza with Rice and Beans		
1 Van de Kamp's Grande Burrito with Rice and Corn		
1 Tyson Chicken Kiev		

Main Meals, Quick and Easy—300 calories

Pick one of these	Plus	Plus one of these
2-ounce beef burger, broiled	1 ounce (dry weight) spaghetti, boiled	2 tablespoons Parmesan cheese
2 breakfast sausage links,	1 medium potato, boiled	1/4 cup baked beans

Pick one of these	Plus	Plus one of these
well grilled and drained	1 small potato, boiled and mashed with skim milk and 1 teaspoon diet margarine	1/2 cup peas
1 fish cake, baked		1/2 cup sweet corn
1 Banquet Gravy with Sliced Beef Entree		1/2 cup beets
2 medium eggs, poached	5 ounces rice, boiled	
6 ounces white fish fillet, grilled, baked, or poached	3 ounces oven fries	
2 ounces ham steak, grilled and well drained	2 2-ounce chunks potato, roasted	
2/3 cup Ragú Meat Sauce	1 burger bun	

3 breakfast sausage links, well grilled and drained	1 small potato, boiled	1/4 cup baked beans
3 fish sticks, baked	1/2 cup noodles, boiled	1/2 cup peas
1 hot dog, boiled	2 ounces oven fries	3 tablespoons sweet corn
1 Mrs. Paul's Crown of Flounder Light Entrée	1/4 cup rice, boiled	1/4 cup lima beans
1 Gorton's Lightly Breaded Fish Fillets	1 hot dog roll	1/4 cup refried beans
	1/2 small pita pocket	

Main Meals, Quick and Easy—400 calories

Pick one of these	*Plus*	*Plus one of these*
1 serving Stouffer's Roast Beef Hash	1 medium potato, boiled	3 tablespoons baked beans
1 Lean Cuisine Veal Primavera	1 small potato, boiled and mashed with skim milk and 1 teaspoon diet margarine	1/3 cup peas
1 Swanson Turkey Entree		1/3 cup sweet corn
1 lamb chop, trimmed, broiled	1/4 cup rice, boiled	1/2 cup green beans
1 pork chop, trimmed, broiled		1/2 cup broccoli
4-ounce rump or fillet steak, well broiled		
1 6-ounce breaded haddock portion, baked, broiled, or dry-fried		
1 chicken breast, baked or broiled, skin removed		
4-ounce ham steak, well broiled		
1 large hot dog, well grilled or dry-fried		
4-ounce fillet of white fish, broiled,		

Pick one of these	Plus	Plus one of these
baked, or dry fried, with 1 portion Cheese Sauce (see recipe, page 259)		
1 Banquet French Chicken Gourmet Entree 1 Banquet Sirloin Tips Supreme Gourmet Entree 2 medium eggs, dry-fried	1/4 cup instant mashed potatoes 1 potato, boiled and mashed with skim milk and 1 teaspoon diet margarine 3 ounces oven fries 2 hash browns 1 medium potato, boiled 1 hot dog roll	1/3 cup peas 1/3 cup sweet corn 1 cup green beans
1 serving Hamburger Helper	1 portion from 50-calorie fruit selection on page 196	

Main Meals, Quick and Easy—500 calories

Pick one of these	Plus	Plus one of these
5-ounce ham steak, grilled	4 ounces oven fries	1/2 cup peas
2 large eggs, dry-fried	1 small potato, baked	1/4 cup baked beans
1 large hot dog, boiled	1 small potato, boiled and sautéed in non-stick pan in 1 teaspoon olive oil	1/2 cup sweet corn
4 breakfast sausage links, grilled and well-drained		1/3 cup lima beans
1 Tyson Chicken Francais Entree	1/4 cup instant mashed potatoes	2 rings pineapple
1 Van de Kamp's Green Chili Beef/Bean Burrito	1 small pita pocket	
1 Swanson Salisbury Steak Main Course Entree		
1 Stouffer's Chicken Divan		
1 Mary Kitchen Corned Beef Hash		
1 Hamburger Helper, any variety		
1 chicken breast, baked or broiled, skin removed		
1 3-ounce cheeseburger		

Pick one of these	*Plus*	*Plus one of these*
1 4-ounce beef-burger, broiled		
5-ounce breaded haddock fillet, baked		
4 fish sticks, baked		
2-egg omelet, cooked in non-stick pan with 1 teaspoon diet margarine and filled with 2 ounces chopped mushrooms		

---

1 Chun King Sweet and Sour Chicken Entree	1 medium potato, boiled	Vegetables or salad from the Unlimiteds list
	3 ounces oven fries	
	1 medium potato, baked	
	1/2 cup rice, boiled	
	1/2 cup refried beans	
	1/4 cup instant mashed potatoes	

Main Meals, Quick and Easy—600 calories

Pick one of these	*Plus*	*Plus one of these*
6-ounce steak, fillet or rump, grilled	5 ounces oven fries	1/2 cup peas
6-ounce ham steak, grilled	6-ounce potato, boiled, sliced, and sautéed in non-stick pan in 1 teaspoon olive oil	1 cup mushrooms, dry-fried
3 ounces liver, plus 2 slices lean, crisp bacon, grilled		1/3 cup baked beans
2 large hot dogs, well grilled		
6-ounce breaded haddock fillet, fried		

---

1 Swanson Beef Pie	4 ounces oven fries	1/4 cup peas
1 Tyson Chicken Jambalaya	4-ounce potato, boiled, sliced, and sautéed in non-stick pan in 1 teaspoon olive oil	1/2 cup green beans
1 Swanson Hungry-Man Turkey Entree		

Main Meals, Heat and Serve—300 calories

Pick one of these	*Plus one of these*
1 Lean Cuisine Oriental Beef with Vegetables and Rice	Any 1 serving from the 25-calorie fruit selection on page 195
1 Lean Cuisine Tuna Lasagna	

Pick one of these   *Plus one of these*

1 Lean Cuisine Veal Primavera
1 Lean Cuisine Fillet of Fish Divan
1 Weight Watchers Chicken Burrito
1 Weight Watchers Southern Fried Chicken Patty
1 Weight Watchers Stuffed Turkey Breast
1 Gorton's Crab Au Gratin
1 Morton's Chicken Chow Mein Light Dinner

---

1 Light and Elegant Beef Teriyaki
1 Weight Watchers Sweet 'n Sour Chicken Tenders
1 Lean Cuisine Fillet of Fish Florentine
1 Lean Cuisine Zucchini Lasagna
1 Lean Cuisine Chicken Chow Mein with Rice
2 Patio Beef Tacos
Franco-American Beef Ravioli in Meat Sauce (7½ ounces)
1 serving Dinty Moore Chicken Stew (7½ ounces)

1 serving from the 50-calorie fruit selection on page 196

---

1 Armour Classic Lite Chicken Burgundy

Any 1 serving from the 50-calorie fruit selec-

Pick one of these	*Plus one of these*
1 Armour Classic Lite Chicken Chow Mein	tion on page 196 plus side salad with oil-free dressing
1 Banquet Macaroni and Cheese (8 ounces)	
1 Chef Boyardee Beef Stew (7 ounces)	
1 Light and Elegant Shrimp Creole	
1 Lean Cuisine Stuffed Cabbage with Meat in Tomato Sauce	

Main Meals, Heat and Serve—400 calories

Pick one of these	*Plus one of these*
1 Weight Watchers Cheese Enchiladas	Any 1 serving from the 25-calorie fruit selection on page 195
1 Armour Dinner Classics Beef Burgundy	
1 Armour Dinner Classics Boneless Beef Short Ribs with Horseradish Sauce	
1 Armour Dinner Classics Sirloin Tips	
1 Banquet Fried Chicken American Dinner	
1 Del Monte Chicken Dinner	
1 Le Menu Yankee Pot Roast	
1 Stouffer's Spaghetti with Meatballs	

---

1 Armour Roast Beef Hash (7½ ounces)	Any 1 serving from the 50-calorie fruit selection on page 196
1 Van de Kamp's Chili with Beans (1 cup)	

Pick one of these   *Plus one of these*

1 Armour Dinner Classics Chicken Milan
1 Armour Dinner Classics Spaghetti with Meatballs
1 Green Giant Chicken and Broccoli with Rice in Cheese Sauce
1 Hormel Sloppy Joe (7 1/2 ounces)
1 Mrs. Smith's Chicken Maison Crepes
1 Stouffer's Beef Chop Suey with Rice
1 Chicken Divan
1 Swanson Swiss Steak

---

1 Weight Watchers Cheese Manicotti
1 Armour Dinner Classics Chicken Tetrazzini
1 Banquet Turkey American Dinner
1 Del Monte Chicken Chow Mein Dinner
1 Le Menu Chicken à la King Dinner
1 Le Menu Ham Steak à la King Dinner
1 Mrs. Smith's Chicken Continental Crepes
1 Swanson Fish 'n Chips

Any 1 serving from the 50 calorie fruit selection on page 196

Main Meals, Heat and Serve—500 calories

Pick one of these

1 Armour Dinner Classics Swedish Meatballs
1 Armour Dinner Classics Boneless Beef Short Ribs with Barbecue Sauce
1 Del Monte Salisbury Steak Dinner
1 Le Menu Chicken Cordon Bleu
1 Le Menu Sliced Breast of Turkey with Mushrooms
1 Patio Cheese Enchilada Dinner
1 Swanson Veal Parmigiana

Plus one of these

Any 1 serving from the 25-calorie fruit selection on page 195

---

1 Armour Dinner Classics Sweet and Sour Chicken
1 Banquet Chicken Pie
1 Green Giant Lasagna with Meat Sauce
1 Le Menu Sweet and Sour Chicken
1 Mrs. Smith's Beef Cannelloni with Tomato Sauce
1 Patio Large Beef and Bean Burrito
1 Stouffer's Spaghetti with Meat Sauce
1 Stouffer's Vegetable Lasagna

Any 1 serving from the 50-calorie fruit selection on page 196

Pick one of these	*Plus one of these*
1 Swanson French Toast with Sausage	
1 Van de Kamp's Cheese Enchilada Dinner	

Pick one of these	*Plus one of these*
1 Armour Corned Beef Hash (7½ ounces)	Any 1 serving from the 50-calorie fruit selection on page 196 plus side salad with oil-free dressing
1 Banquet Chicken with Dumplings Dinner	
1 Banquet Spaghetti and Meatballs Family Favorites	
1 Del Monte Chicken Breast Parmigiana Dinner	
1 Le Menu Chopped Sirloin Beef Dinner	
1 Stouffer's Chicken-Stuffed Pasta Shells with Cheese Sauce	
1 Stouffer's Spinach Crepes with Cheese Sauce	
1 Swanson Scrambled Eggs and Sausage with Hash Brown Potatoes	

Main Meals, Heat and Serve—600 calories

Pick one of these	*Plus one of these*
1 Banquet American Ham Dinner	Any 1 serving from the 50-calorie fruit selection on page 196
1 Banquet American Fish Dinner	
1 Swanson Chunky Beef or Turkey Pie	
1 Van de Kamp's	

Pick one of these   *Plus one of these*

Chicken Suiza with
Rice and Beans
1 Patio Beef Enchilada
Dinner
1 Mrs. Smith's Chicken
Cannelloni with Cheese
Sauce
1 Del Monte Meat Loaf
Dinner
1 Del Monte Beef and
Vegetable Pie
1 Banquet Cheese Enchi-
lada Dinner

Top Takeouts—300 calories*

---

1 McDonald's Hamburger
1 McDonald's Cheeseburger
1 McDonald's Chicken McNuggets (6)
1 McDonald's Egg McMuffin
1 Roy Rogers Roast Beef Sandwich
1 Taco Bell Beef Toastada
1 Burger King Hamburger
1 Burger King Cheeseburger
1 Burger King Whopper, Jr.
1 Arby's Junior Roast Beef
1 Arby's Roasted Chicken Boneless Breast
1 Arby's Roasted Chicken Boneless Leg
1 Arby's Plain Baked Potato
1 Burger King Croissan'wich
1 Church's Fried Chicken Breast
1 Church's Fried Chicken Spicy Nuggets (6)
1 Church's Fried Chicken Catfish Nuggets (4)
1 Dairy Queen Hot Dog

---

* All calories are approximate.

1 Dairy Queen Hot Dog with Chili
1 Jack In The Box Club Pita
1 Jack In The Box Super Taco
1 Kentucky Fried Chicken Original Recipe Side
   Breast or Thigh
1 Kentucky Fried Chicken Kentucky Nuggets

Top Takeouts—400 calories

Choose one of these

1 Arby's Turkey Deluxe
1 Arby's Chicken Salad Sandwich
1 Burger King Whopper, Jr., with Cheese
1 Chick-a-fil Sandwich
1 Chick-a-fil Nuggets
1 Chick-a-fil Hearty Breast of Chicken Soup
1 Dairy Queen Single Burger with Cheese
1 Dairy Queen Fish Fillet
2 Slices Domino's Pepperoni Pizza (12-inch)
2 Slices Domino's Cheese Pizza (16-inch)
1 Hardee's Big Roast Beef Sandwich
1 Hardee's Turkey Club Sandwich
1 Jack In The Box Taco Salad
1 Jack In The Box Pasta Seafood Salad
1 McDonald's Quarterpounder
1 McDonald's Filet-O-Fish
1 McDonald's Sausage McMuffin
1 Roy Rogers Roast Beef Sandwich with Cheese
1 Roy Rogers Large Roast Beef Sandwich
1 Roy Rogers Chicken Breast
1 Roy Rogers Potato with Bacon and Cheese
1 Roy Rogers Egg and Biscuit Platter with Ham
1 Taco Bell Combination Burrito
1 Zantigo Taco Burrito

Top Takeouts—500 calories

Choose one of these

1 Arby's Beef 'n Cheddar
1 Arby's King Roast Beef
1 Arby's Super Roast Beef
1 Arby's Superstuffed Potato, Mushrooms, and
   Cheese
1 Burger King Bacon Double Cheeseburger
1 Burger King Whaler Fish Sandwich
1 Burger King Ham and Cheese Sandwich
1 Burger King Sausage Breakfast Croissan'wich
1 Burger King Scrambled Egg Platter with Bacon
1 Burger King French Toast Sticks
1 Church's Fried Chicken Catfish Nuggets (7)
1 Dairy Queen Double Hamburger
1 Dairy Queen Super Hot Dog
1 Dairy Queen Fish Fillet with Cheese
1 Hardee's 1/4-pound Cheeseburger
1 Hardee's Big Deluxe
1 Hardee's Mushroom n' Swiss Burger
1 Jack In The Box Jumbo Jack
1 Jack In The Box Mushroom Burger
1 McDonald's Quarterpounder with Cheese
1 McDonald's Biscuit with Sausage
1 McDonald's Biscuit with Bacon, Egg, and Cheese
1 McDonald's Sausage McMuffin with Egg
1/2 Pizza Hut Thin-n Crispy Pork Pizza (10-inch)
1/2 Pizza Hut Thin-n Crispy Pizza Supreme (10-
   inch)
1 Roy Rogers Large Roast Beef Sandwich with
   Cheese
1 Roy Rogers Pancake Platter—with syrup, butter,
   bacon

Choose one of these

1 Roy Rogers Pancake Platter—with syrup, butter, ham
1 Taco Bell Beef Burrito
1 Wendy's Big Classic
1 Wendy's Chicken Club
1 Wendy's Broccoli and Cheese Potato
1 Wendy's Chili and Cheese Potato

Top Takeouts—600 calories

Choose one of these

1 Arby's Chicken Breast Sandwich
1 Arby's Chicken Salad with Tomato and Lettuce
1 Arby's Superstuffed Potato Taco
1 Burger King Whopper
2 Church's Fried Chicken Breasts with Wings
1 Dairy Queen Chicken Breast Fillet
1 Jack In The Box Jumbo Jack with Cheese
1 Jack In The Box Chicken Supreme
1 Jack In The Box Sausage Crescent
1 Jack In The Box Pancake Breakfast
1 McDonald's Big Mac
1 McDonald's Biscuit with Sausage and Egg
1/2 Pizza Hut Thick-n Chewy Beef Pizza (10-inch)
1 Roy Rogers RR Bar Burger
1 Roy Rogers Bacon Cheeseburger
1 Roy Rogers Chicken Breast and Wing
1 Roy Rogers Pancake Platter—with syrup, butter, sausage
1 Wendy's Double Burger with Cheese

Choose one of these

1 Wendy's Bacon and Cheese Potato
1 Wendy's Cheese Potato

Top Takeouts—700 calories

Choose one of these

1 Burger King Whopper with Cheese
1 Burger King Chicken Sandwich
1 Burger King Scrambled Egg Platter with Sausage
1 Dairy Queen Triple Hamburger
4 Slices Domino's Cheese Pizza (12-inch)
1 Jack In The Box Bacon Cheeseburger Supreme
1 Jack In The Box Sirloin Steak Dinner
1 Jack In The Box Shrimp Dinner
1 Jack In The Box Nachos Supreme
1 Jack In The Box Scrambled Eggs Breakfast
1 McDonald's McDLT
1/2 Pizza Hut Thick-n Chewy Pizza Supreme (10-inch)
1 Wendy's Big Double Classic

Cooked Vegetables, Pasta and Rice—25 calories

Choose one of these

1/2 cup green beans
1/3 cup beets
1/2 cup broccoli
1/2 cup carrots
1 cup zucchini

Choose one of these

1/2 cup cooked mixed, chopped vegetables
1/2 cup stewed tomatoes

Vegetables, Pasta, and Rice—50 calories

Choose one of these

1/4 cup mixed bean salad
1/4 cup lima beans
2/3 cup snow-pea pods
1/2 cup parsnips
1/2 cup green peas
1/2 cup new potatoes
1 cup spinach
1/3 cup corn
1/4 cup refried beans
1/2 cup green beans with almonds

Vegetables, Pasta, and Rice—75 calories

Choose one of these

1/2 cup red kidney beans
1/2 cup winter squash
2 fried onion rings
1/2 cup pickled beets
3 ounces hash brown potatoes

Vegetables, Pasta, and Rice—100 calories

Choose one of these

1 small baked potato
1/4 cup hash browns
1/2 cup lima beans
1/4 cup baked beans
1/2 cup three-bean salad
1/2 cup boiled rice
1 baked sweet potato
1/2 cup canned sweet potato
1/2 cup egg noodles
1/2 cup potato salad
1/2 cup scalloped potatoes
1/2 cup creamed onions
1/2 cup creamed spinach
1/2 cup creamed corn
1 ear corn

Vegetables, Pasta, and Rice—150 calories

Choose one of these

1/4 cup prepared instant mashed potatoes
3 ounces oven fries
3 ounces potato puffs
1/3 cup hash browns
1 medium baked potato
1/2 cup rice pilaf
1/2 cup fried rice
1/2 cup chow mein noodles

Fruits and Juices—25 calories

Fruits can be fresh, frozen, cooked (if using sugar, this must be taken from your Treats allowance), or canned and drained (weights are given for the drained fruit).

2 fresh apricots
1/3 cup blackberries
1/2 cup raspberries
1 small tangerine
1/2 cup strawberries
1 small plum
1/3 cup tomato juice
1 cup rhubarb

Fruits and Juices—50 calories

Fruits can be fresh, frozen, cooked (if using sugar, this must be taken from your Treats allowance), or canned and drained (weights are given for the drained fruits).

1/4 cup apple juice
3 drained apricot halves
10 cherries
1/2 cup grapefruit sections
1/2 medium grapefruit
1 kiwi fruit
15 grapes
1 small nectarine
1 peach or 1/4 cup peach slices, drained
1/2 cup fresh pineapple
1/2 cup orange juice

1/2 cup apple juice
1/3 cup pineapple juice
1/2 cup fruit salad
1/2 cup mandarin orange sections
1 cup watermelon

Fruits and Juices—100 calories

1/2 cup apple sauce
1 apple
1 pear
5 dates
1 banana
1 pomegranate
1 orange

Milk and Yogurt—50 calories

2/3 cup skim milk
1/2 cup low-fat milk
1/3 cup whole milk

Milk and Yogurt—100 calories

---

1 1/4 cups skim milk
1 cup low-fat milk (1%)
2/3 cup whole milk
1 8-ounce container plain non-fat yogurt

Treats, Snacks, and Extras—25 calories

Sweet Treats

1 heaping teaspoon sugar
2 level teaspoons marmalade, jam, or honey

1 cube sugar
3 Lifesavers
1 fortune cookie

Savory Treats/Extras

2 tablespoons bread-and-butter pickles
1/4 cup taco sauce
1/4 cup salsa
1 pat butter
1 crispbread
2 Melba toast rounds
1 teaspoon mayonnaise
1 tablespoon reduced-calorie salad dressing

Treats, Snacks, and Extras—50 calories

Sweet Treats

1 package sugar-free hot-cocoa mix
2 Nabisco's Socials tea cookies 1 Keebler's fudge
stripe cookies
2 gingersnaps
2 honey grahams
1 Weight Watchers yogurt

Savory Treats

1 breakfast sausage link, well grilled
1 slice lean ham
1 tablespoon tartar sauce
1 taco shell
1 cup unbuttered popcorn

Extras

1/2 tablespoon butter or margarine
1 tablespoon heavy or whipped cream
2 tablespoons sour cream
1 tablespoon reduced-calorie mayonnaise

Drinks

1 can alcohol-free lager

Treats, Snacks, and Extras—75 calories

Sweet Treats

1 Oreo cookie
2 Kraft chocolate fudgies
15 chocolate-covered raisins
Any three sweet treats from 25-calorie list, or one from 25-calorie and one from 50-calorie list.

Savory Treats

1 slice bread
2 malted-milk peanut-butter sandwich crackers
12 Cheez-It crackers
2 rice crackers

Extras

Any three extras from 25-calorie list, or one from 25-calorie and one from 50-calorie list.

Treats, Snacks, and Extras—100 calories

Sweet Treats

6 ounces Grape, Orange, or Apple Crush
1/2 Charleston Chew!
10 Junior Mints
2 KitKat fingers
12 animal crackers
2 Fig Newtons
1 Stella D'Oro Breakfast Treat
2 chocolate graham crackers
2 Pepperidge Farm Irish Oatmeal cookies
1 Tastykake chocolate cupcake
1 Hostess Ho-ho
1 Drake's Yodels

Sweet Treats—Desserts

1/2 cup custard
1/2 cup sugar-free pudding
1 juice bar
1/2 cup sorbet
1/2 cup frozen yogurt
1/2 cup ice milk

Drinks

1 bottle light beer
1 5-ounce glass dry red or white wine, or champagne
1 1/2 ounces liquor with calorie-free mixer (optional)

Extras

1 slice bread with 1 teaspoon diet margarine
1 tablespoon butter
2 tablespoons diet margarine
1/2 cup boiled or 1 small baked potato
1 tablespoon mayonnaise
1 medium egg, dry-fried
2 ounces lean meat
2 ounces oven fries

Treats, Snacks, and Extras—150 calories

Sweet Treats

1 Baby Ruth bar, 1 ounce
1/2 Butterfinger bar
14 chocolate-covered peanuts
1 Cadbury Fruit and Nut bar
1 Hostess Twinkie
1 package Little Debbie Golden Cremes
1 package Little Debbie Fudge or Coconut Rounds
1 Carnation Chocolate Fudge Heaven Sunday bar
2/3 cup vanilla ice cream

Savory Treats

1 ounce Cheddar cheese and 1 crispbread
1 ounce bag potato chips
1 ounce bag corn chips
1 ounce bag cheese popcorn
4 cups microwave popcorn

Drinks

1 can regular beer
1 can regular soda

Treats, Snacks, and Extras—200 calories

Sweet Treats

1 Pillsbury turnover
1 Sara Lee Pound Cake snack cake
1 Nabisco Toastettes
1 serving Sara Lee Cheese Cake
1 serving Sara Lee Deluxe Carrot Cake
8 Hershey's Kisses
1 Planters peanut bar
1 package Sugar Babies
3 Pepperidge Farm Brussels cookies
2 molasses cookies
6 Pepperidge Farm Orleans cookies
1 small muffin

Sweet Treats—Desserts and Ice Cream

1 cup ice milk
1 low-fat fruit yogurt
1 Good Humor Fudge Cake
1/2 cup ice cream

Savory Treats

1 ounce mixed nuts
1 1/2 ounces peanuts
1 1/2 ounces tortilla chips with salsa

Treats, Snacks, and Extras—250 calories

Sweet Treats

1 Blueberry Muffin
1 McDonald's Apple Pie
5 Fig Newtons

5 Duncan Hines Chocolate Chip Cookies
4 Almost Home Fudge Chocolate Chip Cookies
12 Ginger Snaps
1 Hershey Bar None
1 Hershey Milk Chocolate with Almonds (1.55 oz)
1 Peanut M&Ms (1.7 oz)

Sweet Treats—Desserts and Ice Cream

1 ice cream sandwich
1 Oreo Cookies 'n Cream Sandwich
1/2 cup Häagen Dazs Vanilla
1 cup Baskin-Robbins Vanilla Frozen Yogurt
1/2 cup Ben & Jerry's French Vanilla
1 Good Humor Full O'Chocolate
1 cup Dole Pineapple Sorbet

Savory Treats

1 ear of corn with butter
2 slices Domino's 10" Mushroom Sausage Pizza
1 regular fries
1 Jack-in-the-Box Fajita Pita
1 McDonald's Hamburger
21/2-oz Cheddar Cheese
15 Ritz Crackers
11/2-oz bar-B-Que Potato Chips

❖ 9. ❖

Eating Out—
and Days Off

IT IS A RARE DIET BOOK THAT TREATS DIETERS LIKE OR-
dinary human beings who actually want to do normal things occasionally, like go out for a meal, visit
friends for dinner, or even take a vacation.

However, I know that you do have a life $B > D >$
(beyond diet), and if I don't recognize that fact, your
dieting success will suffer.

Every year $215 billion is spent (and the amount
is rising) on eating out in the U.S.: $17.25 for every
man, woman, and child every week. In reality,
though, we're divided into two groups—people who
eat out very frequently, usually because of their
work; and people who eat out only occasionally, usually for social reasons. Depending upon which group
you fall into, we have to apply different tactics.

FREQUENT FEASTING

Let's be realistic. If you are in the habit of eating
out every day (or nearly every day), be it a truck
stop or a five-star restaurant, there's no point in my
telling you that you can eat as much as you want
and still lose weight. These meals have probably
been the very reason you put on weight in the first

place, and trying to diet around them is going to be almost impossible. The reasons are these:

- Chefs, whether they are of the egg-and-hash brigade or the haute-cuisine school, rarely give a thought to how many calories their concoctions contain. Diner and cafeteria meals are often high in surplus fat that you would have avoided had you been cooking the same meals yourself The Junk Food Diet way. Continental and upscale eating places tend to provide everything coated with rich sauces or swamped in butter.
- Restaurants need to make a profit—and they stand more of a chance of doing that if you eat three courses rather than one. Add to that the temptation of "free" food such as rolls and butter, or after-dinner sweets, or chips with a sandwich, etc., and it's so easy to eat far more than you ever intended.
- Portion sizes are often large, especially in diners. So, even if what you have on your plate isn't a particularly high-calorie food, the amount you're given turns it into a high-calorie plateful.
- Your own natural greed. If you are eating at home and three-quarters of the way through the meal you have had enough, you will probably leave the rest. In a restaurant, you are much more likely to think, "If I've paid for it, I'm damned well going to eat it." And how about if someone else is paying? Then the temptation to eat all you can is even stronger.
- If you eat out, you drink.

So my first question for you to ponder is: Are all these meals out really necessary? Could you not take a brown-bag lunch to work instead, or on the road, if you have to travel? Could you not get by with a takeout sandwich at this time of day, and have a big meal when you get home in the evening?

If you come to the conclusion that there genuinely is no way around your eating-out dilemma, then what we have to do is attempt to bring the calorie content of all those meals down to an acceptable level within your diet.

First, then, here are some general guidelines for you to follow:

- Follow the Pick Your Own Plan rather than the Set Diet, and treat your meal out as your main meal of the day.
- If you have a choice of where to eat, go somewhere that has several items on its menu that are plain, straightforward dishes in which it is hard to "hide" calories. On a daily basis, for instance, Chinese, Italian, and French restaurants are lethal.
- Always keep The Junk Food Diet rules in your mind when you're eating out. For instance, cut visible fat off meat and stop eating when you're full.
- If possible, pick a restaurant that will allow you to have your vegetables without butter—your "grilled" fish really grilled and not coated in butter.
- Eat your fill of plain cooked vegetables or salad, and again, ask for them all ungarnished or without sauces or dressing. Remember, not all vegetables are low in calories—fried onion rings, mushrooms, eggplant, zucchini, and all kinds of fried potatoes are high in calories.

- Try some forward planning. Decide what you're going to eat beforehand if possible so you needn't be tempted by the menu descriptions.
- Use your common sense. Despite all my warnings, you can eat a reasonable dieter's meal in any restaurant if you're sensible. Just remember that the most fattening foods are fats, and things containing fat, such as pastry, oily sauces like mayonnaise and hollandaise, vinaigrette, and deep-fried small items like shoe-string fries. However, a little of one or two high-calorie items is probably all right. Use your common sense!

Armed with these guidelines, here's what you do next. You'll remember that your main meal should be not more than 500 calories if you're on 1,000 calories a day, or 600 calories if you're dieting on 1,250 or 1,500 calories a day. With the help of the meal listings at the end of this chapter, you simply pick your meal to the correct total, or less. Then make sure that the rest of what you eat on the same day doesn't add up to more than your allowed calorie total.

If you want to use your daily Treats calories on an "extra" with your meal, such as a drink, a dessert, or some butter, then do so—but remember, you'll be leaving yourself with not many calories left for the rest of the day.

You will find it hard to pick a three-course meal in a restaurant and still stay within your 500- or 600-calorie limit. I don't believe you really need three courses, anyway, but you could, if you are determined, have a dessert as your daily Treat.

The only way you can be really sure that you're

doing okay is to ask yourself the pertinent question: Am I still losing weight?

INFREQUENT FEASTING

Celebrations are what make life worthwhile. Whether it's a birthday, a wedding, a new job, or a holiday—everyone needs something to celebrate now and then. But a celebration means food and drink.

At such times, there is only one thing worse than having to say, "Sorry, I can't eat that/drink that/come out with you—I'm on a diet," and that is hearing someone else say it instead. When people want to have a good time, diet bores are deadly.

So the next time that happens to you, don't even think about sticking to your diet. I give you permission to eat what you want without feeling guilty. And that's important. If you feel guilty, not only will you not enjoy yourself, but you'll also feel so bad afterward that you'll abandon your diet.

The reason there is no need to feel guilty is that I have a very simple way for you to indulge without ruining your diet. It's a system called the Treats Transfer.

Treats transfer

Why is it that when you sit down for a meal with a friend, you eat less than she does, and yet she is thin and you are not?

It is probably quite simply that she, without even thinking about it, obeys the first law of eating: balance. She'll eat trillions of calories tonight, but tomorrow she may eat very little. In other words, she quite naturally practices the calorie common sense that overweight people tend to ignore.

You must learn not to ignore it—and by practicing the Treats Transfer, you can. Here's how it works.

Fact one: Whichever calorie level you're dieting on, you have a daily Treats allowance of either 100, 150, or 250 calories a day. Fact two: If you're going out somewhere special for a meal or party or day out, you almost always know well in advance.

All you have to do is cut down a little on your food intake for a while before your special event by "saving" those Treats calories rather than "spending" (eating) them.

Now, although you may not know exactly what you're going to eat at your celebration, I can tell you that at any one meal, if you are an "average" person, you will eat not more than 1,500 calories at most. You may get through it with far less, even including alcohol. On the other hand, you may know exactly what you will eat—for instance, that you will have, if it's available, shrimp cocktail, plus bread, chicken Kiev, and Black Forest cake, together with a few glasses of wine. Now, I can tell you from looking up the lists I compiled at the end of this chapter, those few things come to around 1,400 calories.

Now, say you're on the 1,250 calorie-a-day diet. On the day you are due to go out for this meal, you have a 200-calorie breakfast and a 300-calorie lunch, plus 100 calories for fruit and milk. That leaves you with 650 calories left toward your evening out, which means you have to find an extra 750 calories from somewhere. Easy! All you do is forgo your daily Treat of 150 calories a day for five days beforehand. Then you can go out, eat your favorite meal, drink your wine, and not need to feel one tiny bit guilty, because you know you aren't doing any damage to your diet. Good, isn't it?

You try some more possible combinations yourself. Make up some meals you'd really like, work out how many surplus calories you need to borrow, and see how few days it takes for you to "earn" them. It's a very reassuring pastime.

You can use the Treats Transfer in other ways: for an ice cream out while shopping with friends, or a whole day off your diet every Sunday, say. All you ever have to do is work out roughly what your night or day "off" is going to "cost" and allow for it. It's always best to "save up" in advance, rather than trying to pay back your calorie bank after the event. Paying for something after you've had it is always harder; the incentive of having something to look forward to has gone.

I would also suggest that you practice the Treats Transfer as an occasional thing—no more than once a week; otherwise, you'll get confused with your figures. And once you get confused, you are likely to start cheating.

How do you know you're doing okay? If you're losing weight, you're doing all right.

CHRISTMAS AND HOLIDAYS

Last, a word or two about celebrations that go on longer than an evening or a day . . . your annual vacation, say, or Christmas.

My advice is for you to treat yourself like a normal person, and behave like one, which means eating what you like in moderation most of the time, having the odd blowout, and also having times when you can leave food alone because there's something better going on.

Think of food as part of your break/holiday, not the be-all and end-all of it.

If you try the alternative, sticking to your diet while everyone around you is eating, drinking, and being merry, you're handing yourself a recipe for disaster—a battle on your plate.

With a relaxed attitude, okay, you may put on a couple of pounds during the break; you certainly won't lose much. But afterward you can get back to steady weight loss with no real damage done.

Eating-Out Guide

(All calorie counts are approximate for standard restaurant-sized servings, unless stated otherwise)

Cafeteria or Diner

2 eggs over easy, home fries, bacon, toast	655
1 burger with fries	535
2 hot dogs and fries	530
2 pork chops, corn, and mashed potatoes	575
plain omelet with salad and dressing	425
plain omelet and fries	450
ham-salad sandwich	300
quiche and salad	455
egg-salad sandwich	440
pot pie, vegetables	600

meat loaf	450
beef stew and roll with salad	350

Lunch Counter or Deli

English muffin with jelly	232
ham and Swiss on rye	650
tuna-salad sandwich	350
grilled cheese	500
chicken salad sandwich	310
club sandwich	470
potato salad	180
macaroni salad	180
coleslaw	50
Ruben sandwich	550
pastrami on rye	475
roast-beef sandwich	350

Italian Restaurant

lasagna	450
spaghetti with meatballs	800
cannelloni or manicotti	700
garlic-butter-stuffed chicken with vegetables	800
tagliatelle with cream and ham	400
veal scallops with vegetables	600
garlic bread	180
tortellini with meat	500
chicken cacciatore	790
minestrone soup	200
mozzarella cheese and tomato salad	250
risotto	600
spaghetti with meat sauce	600
spaghetti with tomato sauce	450

fettuccine Alfredo	910
angel hair pasta with plum-tomato-and-basil sauce	470
spaghetti with pesto sauce	880
linguine with red clam sauce	490
linguine with white clam sauce	660
ravioli with meat sauce	610

Greek Restaurant

taramasalata, 2-ounce serving	270
hummus, 2-ounce serving	100–150
1 pita pocket	180
stuffed vine leaves as an appetizer (3 leaves)	150–200
stuffed vine leaves with rice (main course)	600
1 lamb kebab stick with vegetables and rice	450
1 average portion baked lamb and salad	400
1 Greek salad with feta cheese, including olive oil	250
moussaka, 14 ounces	770

Chinese Restaurant

barbecued spare ribs	400
shark's fin soup	90
chicken chop suey	400
chicken chow mein	400
1/4 of an average set Chinese meal for 4	900

Mexican Restaurant

1 taco	180
enchiladas, average serving	380
1 bean burrito	360
steak fajita	235
Mexican pizza	715
nachos	356
chili	430
taco salad	900
guacamole, average serving	130
refried beans	330

Salad Bar

3 cups lettuce	20
1/2 cup cottage cheese	110
1/4 cup turkey or ham	50
1/4 cup cheese	90
2 breadsticks	35
1/2 cup alfalfa sprouts	10
1/4 cup peppers	15
4 slices cucumber	10
1/4 cup mushrooms	10
1/4 cup radishes	10
1/4 cup tomatoes	10
1 ladle bacon bits	10
1 ladle chow mein noodles	70
1 ladle croutons	60
1 tablespoon chopped egg	30
2 tablespoons Parmesan cheese	130
2 tablespoons sunflower seeds and raisins	140
1 ladle dressing	130
1 ladle reduced-calorie dressing	100

Steak House

8-ounce prime rib	575
4-ounce prime rib	285
6-ounce sirloin	650
4-ounce sirloin tip	235
6-ounce filet mignon	330
7-ounce rib eye	665
steak sandwich	375
baked potato with butter	245
french fries	230
side salad without dressing	30
6-ounce chopped steak	460
8-ounce sirloin	900
8-ounce T-bone	1045
13-ounce T-bone	1612
steak fries	425
peppers and onions	80
mushroom sauce	25

Doughnut Shop and Bakery

glazed jelly doughnut	300
plain doughnut	200
doughnut hole	50
iced chocolate doughnut	210
glazed doughnut	210
chocolate croissant	550
plain croissant	300
brownie	280
chocolate chip cookie	130
bran muffin	355
corn muffin	350
blueberry muffin	275

bagel, plain	250
danish pastry	235

Fast-Food Restaurants

McDonald's

(Calorie counts are exact)

Hamburger (regular)	263
Cheeseburger	318
Quarterpounder	427
McDLT	600
Quarterpounder with Cheese	525
Big Mac	570
Filet-O-Fish	435
Chicken McNuggets (6)	323
Chicken McNuggets (9)	485
barbecue sauce	60
sweet-and-sour sauce	64
hot mustard sauce	63
french fries, regular	220
french fries, large	312
apple pie	253
vanilla milk shake	354
chocolate milk shake	388
big breakfast	642
Bacon and Egg McMuffin	311
Sausage and Egg McMuffin	451
Egg McMuffin	293
biscuit with sausage	440
hot cakes with butter and syrup	413
McDonaldland cookies	288
side salad	57
chicken salad Oriental	141

shrimp salad	104
hash browns	131
scrambled eggs	157

Burger King

(calorie counts are exact)

Bacon Double Cheeseburger	510
Cheeseburger	317
Chicken in a Bun	688
Whaler sandwich	488
Hamburger	275
Whopper	863
Whopper with Cheese	945
french fries, regular	227
onion rings	274
apple pie	305
milk shake	340
french toast sticks	499

Pizza Hut

Thin-n Crispy Beef (1/2 10-inch pie)	490
Thin-n Crispy Pork (1/2 10-inch pie)	520
Thin-n Crispy Cheese (1/2 10-inch pie)	450
Thin-n Crispy Pepperoni (1/2 10-inch pie)	430
Thin-n Crispy Supreme (1/2 10-inch pie)	510
Thick 'n Chewy Beef (1/2 10-inch pie)	620
Thick 'n Chewy Pork (1/2 10-inch pie)	640
Thick 'n Chewy Cheese (1/2 10-inch pie)	560

Thick 'n Chewy Pepperoni (1/2 10-inch pie)	560
Thick 'n Chewy Supreme (1/2 10-inch pie)	640

Kentucky Fried Chicken

Original Recipe

wing	180
side breast	275
center breast	257
drumstick	150
thigh	275

Extra Crispy

wing	220
side breast	355
center breast	355
drumstick	175
thigh	370

6 nuggets	275
buttermilk biscuits	270
mashed potato with gravy	60
chicken gravy	60
Kentucky fries	270
coleslaw	100
potato salad	140
baked beans	100
corn on the cob	175

Long John Silver's

Fish and Fries, 3 pieces fish	853
Fish and Fries, 2 pieces fish	650

Fish and More with slaw, 2 hush puppies	978
Fish Dinner with slaw, 2 hush puppies, fries	1180
Shrimp, Fish, or Chicken Dinner with fries, slaw, 2 hush puppies	1022
Seafood Platter	976
Clam Dinner	955
Battered Shrimp Dinner	711
Scallop Dinner	747
Baked Fish Dinner	387
Shrimp Salad	183
Seafood Salad	406
Ocean Chef's Salad	222
clam chowder	128

SUMMARY OF WHAT YOU'VE READ IN CHAPTER 9

- If you eat out regularly, you need to recognize that these meals should be controlled.
- You can get a reasonably low-calorie meal almost anywhere if you really want to.
- If you eat out infrequently, go ahead and enjoy yourself.
- Don't bother dieting on vacation.

❧ 10. ❧

Success!
Now Stay Thin
for Life

WELL DONE! YOU LOST THOSE EXTRA POUNDS WITH your own determination (and a little help from me), so you have every right to feel pleased with yourself. It wasn't that hard, was it?

Now comes the part that's even more important: *staying thin*.

It is a fact that most people find keeping the weight off harder than losing it. It is a fact that two-thirds of dieters put some or all of their weight back on sooner or later. For most, it's within a year of losing it.

What a terrible waste of effort! I want to make sure you are not one of those people.

PRACTICALITIES

To begin with, let's deal with the immediate, pleasant task of getting you off your low-calorie diet and back on to a non-dieting, but non-fattening, one.

Thanks to The Junk Food Diet, two of the most common problems dieters face when they come back to a normal diet won't apply to you.

First, be glad you didn't follow a fad diet—a liquids-only diet, say, or a grapefruit-and-fish diet, for
example. Those are the diets that do nothing whatsoever for you in the long term, because they don't
teach you long-term sensible eating habits that you
can live with. Having lost weight on The Junk Food
Diet, you will easily make the transition back to a
normal diet because "normal" will be almost identi-
cal to the weight-loss one—only there will be more
of it. . . .

Second, be glad you didn't crash-diet—lose weight
too quickly. It's a fact that weight lost quickly
comes back quickly. On The Junk Food Diet, you
had plenty to eat and you lost weight gradually.

So, with those two pluses, you have a head start
in the staying-thin game. Now, how best to cash in?
First, I'll explain a couple of things you should
know about what happens when you start eating
more after a period of eating less.

And, remember when you began dieting how I explained to you that three pounds or so of the initial,
high, first week's weight loss would be fluid, not fat?
Well, when you step up your food intake, the fluid
levels in your body also adjust, but this time you
gain fluid (and carbohydrates) rather than lose it.
You may, indeed, gain those three pounds back
again. This is not fat, it is fluid. It is the same fluid
that causes people to say, guiltily and almost unbe-
lievingly, after they've eaten just one big meal, "I've
gained weight!" To a point, the more carbohydrates
you eat, the more fluid your body retains. It's normal, healthy functioning. In other words, if you finish dieting at, say, 125 pounds, the fluid increase
will mean you level out at between 128 and 130
pounds. However, because of the way we're going to

get you up to your maintenance diet level, this fluid gain won't be an overnight thing. It will be gradual. And, because we will be building up your calorie level gradually, too, you will find that you probably lose another pound or two of fat before we get you up to maintenance over the next six weeks or so—so that the extra fat loss will balance out the fluid gain and you'll still end up 125 pounds (or whatever).

One thing you should know is that people who tell you they have to stay on a strict low-calorie diet for life in order to stay thin are exaggerating grossly.

Unless you're foolishly trying to maintain a weight that's far too low for your height, that just isn't true. On the other hand, it is true to say that you can't go back to eating as much as you did when you were overweight. This is for two reasons. One, eating that much made you fat. Eating that much again will make you fat again. Two, remember, I explained to you that a 225-pound man needs more to eat than a 125-pound woman to maintain his weight. And you, at, say, 125 pounds, need less food to maintain your new size than you did at, say, 155 pounds (unless, of course, you keep your exercise level up).

So please don't feel cheated that you can't go back to eating however much it was that you were eating before this diet.

What you will be able to do is eat a reasonably normal amount for a person of normal weight. According to the Recommended Dietary Allowance for an average woman between nineteen and fifty carrying out most occupations, you need around 2,000 calories a day to maintain normal body weight, but the figure varies from 1,600 up to 2,500 for different age groups and levels of activity. Men in most occupations between ages nineteen and twenty-two need around 2,900 calories a day, and men between twenty-three and fifty need 2,700—but again, the figures for men of different age groups and occupations vary from 2,000 up to 3,300.

What all this means is that although it is likely that you will need somewhere around 2,000 calories a day if you are female or 2,700 to 2,900 if you're male, these figures are only a guide. Everyone is different, and just as you lost on the level that was right for you, so your maintenance level will be specific to you and may be different from your friend's.

So please don't feel too badly if you happen to be the woman or man who needs fewer calories than your next-door neighbor. What other people eat is no concern of yours. You must eat what you need for your own body.

If you are one of the minority of people who don't need many calories a day—say you find your maintenance level is only 1,700—you can, if you wish, speed up your metabolic rate (your calorie-consuming system) with a few crafty tactics. You can step up the amount of aerobic exercise you do—walking, cycling, and so on. You can build up the amount of muscle in your body (by a daily workout with light weights, for instance), because muscle burns up calories more readily than other body tissue does.

But, looking on the positive side, even if you do need slightly fewer calories than your friend, the fact is that you can still eat more than when you were dieting without getting fat again. Considerably more. Anybody who says otherwise is not telling the truth. What we have to do is discover what that amount is.

THE TRANSITION PERIOD

Because neither you nor I can predict your calorie-maintenance requirements exactly, the only safe way to start eating more is to build up your food intake gradually. Here, step by step, is what you do.

Week One

Whatever you do, do not get on the scales, say "Yippee! I did it!," and go on a week-long binge. If you do, you'll have wasted the very considerable asset your diet has given you: the fact that less is now normal. You are used to smaller amounts; don't give your stomach or your brain the chance to get back into the habit of eating a lot more right away.

Instead, do this: Whatever dieting calorie level you finished on, add 250 calories, so that each day this week you eat 1,250 if you were on 1,000; 1,500 if you were on 1,250; and 1,750, if by any chance, you finished your diet still on 1,500 calories. (If you did, you're probably male.) Continue as before, picking your food from the listings in Chapter 8. Make sure the extra calories aren't Sweet Treats, though. Stick to your new calorie level throughout Week One. You may notice a small FLUID weight gain (say, 1–1½ lbs).

Weeks Two and Three

Add another 250 calories to your diet. For these two weeks, your level will now be either 1,500, 1,750, or 2,000, again made up from the meal choices in the Pick Your Own listings, but not from the Sweet

Treats. As you increase your total daily calorie level, it's best to keep your Treats/Extra allowance to a maximum of 250 calories a day. (See pages 197–202.)

A further small weight gain due to fluid may occur. Nobody I know of will yet have reached the stage where he or she is gaining FAT weight. (If you are on 2,000 calories a day now, it is because you were still losing on 1,500).

Weeks Four and Five

Add on another 250 calories. So for these two weeks, you will be on either 1,750, 2,000, or 2,250 calories a day. A few of you may have reached your maintenance level by now, but this won't become obvious until Week Six. Fluid gain should have ceased.

Week Six—onward

Now start adding in blocks of 100 calories more each week. So for Week Six you are on either 1,850, 2,100, or 2,350 calories a day. Week Seven you are on 1,950, 2,200, or 2,450, and so on. At this stage you should weigh yourself once a week at the same time of day with no clothes on, on the same scale. If there's no weight gain (assuming, for women, you aren't pre-period), add another 100 calories for another week, and then weigh yourself again.

Sooner or later (it will probably be sooner now), you will get on the scale and find you've put on half a pound or a pound. This will not be fluid; it will be fat. That means that you've passed your maintenance level, and it's time to go back to the level you were on the previous week. Say you've spent a week on 2,200 calories a day and you've gained; go back to 2,100. That is your permanent maintenance level.

This is not to say that you should eat exactly 2,100 calories every day for the rest of your life. Some days you will eat a bit more, some a bit less; some weeks you'll eat more, some less. But if you average out at that amount over a period of time, you will never put on weight again—except by getting much older (we need about 50 calories a day less for every five years older we get over the age of thirty).

Don't skip doing this climbing up to your maintenance level. I repeat, levels vary so much from person to person that I can't tell you what yours will be. What you want is control of the situation—and this way, you have it.

YOUR MAINTENANCE DIET

Having found your correct daily calorie level, you can stick to it simply by following The Junk Food Diet principles. Just pick a wide variety of meals and foods from the listings in Chapter 8, up to your new calorie level. When shopping, look for calorie information on the labels for the convenience foods you buy. You can buy a comprehensive calorie counter.

Remember, the tips that helped you to lose are the ones that will help you stay thin; don't waste calories on high-calorie foods when low-calorie ones will do just as well; and don't forget those crafty ways to cut the fat out of your diet.

I'm not saying you should spend the rest of your life counting calories. Far from it. But if you keep an eye on what you eat, bearing in mind your known calorie maintenance level, you won't get fat again.

Here are some more tips to help you stay thin and healthy:

- Eat a varied diet.
- Don't eat mindlessly: Be aware of what you're eating and always ask yourself, "Do I really need this?"
- Let hunger be your main reason for eating.
- Several small snacks a day rather than a few big meals will keep you from ever getting too hungry and will help increase your metabolic rate.
- Put small to medium portions on your plate rather than big ones. For instance, if you're serving potatoes and are not sure whether to give yourself two pieces or three, have two. If you're still genuinely hungry at the end of your meal, you can always have some more.
- Smaller plate and dish sizes will help you control your portion sizes.
- Build your favorite foods into your diet so that you never feel deprived.
- Eat slowly. If you eat too fast, you'll tend to finish your meal still feeling falsely hungry. That's where foods that need some chewing, like fiber-rich vegetables, help.
- Never let yourself get so hungry that you'll eat anything and everything in sight.
- Continue with The Junk Food Diet policy on Sweet Treats: Have no more than 250 calories' worth a day, or 2,100 a week.
- Weigh yourself once a week, no more, no less, at the same time of day with no clothes on, on the same scale.

So there you have all the practical advice you really need to stay thin forever. But you're only human, and I would like to forewarn you with some sensible advice on what to do should the unthinkable happen and you find you have put on a little weight.

THE THIN END OF THE WEDGE

For most of us, weight slips back on gradually. We lead busy lives, perhaps we stop being quite so careful with our diet during a particularly busy time, perhaps we don't weigh ourselves for a while—and then we discover the truth. In fact, we might have put on so much weight that it's diet time again, and what a daunting prospect it can be the second time around!

This is exactly what I want you to avoid. So I want you to promise me that, without getting obsessive about it, you will weigh yourself once a week, after what you consider a normal day's eating—not after a celebration blowout, for instance (and, for women, not just before a period).

If you get on the scale at this weekly weigh-in and find you have put on a couple of pounds, don't panic. And don't despair. That sounds like a fat person's thinking. And you're not a fat person.

No, what you do is remember that you're a normal person. And what do normal people do when they have put on a couple of pounds? They cut back a little for a day or two, and lose it. So that's what you do.

If you need the security of a regulated plan, then go back on The Junk Food Diet—1,500-calorie level, either the Set Diet or the Pick Your Own Plan—for around a week.

If you don't need that much structure, simply put small portions of the higher-calorie foods on your plate and make up the spaces with bigger portions of the lower-calorie ones.

What you don't want to do is ignore that couple of pounds, hoping they'll go away of their own accord. They won't. Again, that's a fat person's thinking. Unless you do something about the extra pounds now, what they will do is cunningly turn into ten pounds. If you decide you can live with the extra weight for a while, that pound or two will be nearer ten, and at some stage you will have to make the decision: Do I diet again or go on getting fatter?

You should never put on more than three or four pounds without doing something about it right away.

If I have to pick the single most important factor that will help you to stay thin for life without hassle, it's this: Don't let yourself get more than a few pounds over the weight you feel best at, ever. Anything more is the thin end of the wedge.

BEING A SLIM PERSON

I leave you with some last words of advice, which I hope you won't need. There are some people, probably a lot more than you'd imagine, who never really feel like thin people even if they succeed in dieting. This doesn't happen just to very obese people or to people who have been seriously overweight for years. It can also happen to people who always want to be 15 pounds or so less than they are.

It's a great temptation, if you've been plagued in

one way or another by your weight for years, to feel that even though you've lost weight this time, your size is beyond your control. You know what to do to stay thin, but you don't do it. Somewhere deep down you feel that your larger size is the real you, your slim self an impostor.

So listen—you aren't a fat person wearing a temporarily thin body. You *are* a thin person. When you were fat you were a thin person in a fat person's body. And don't let anyone tell you otherwise. (I've known successful dieters who really did put weight back on again because jealous friends or selfish relatives persuaded them to.)

So please remember that you, and only you, are responsible for your own size. You weren't meant to be fat; no one is meant to be fat. You can't alter your natural height, your frame size, or even a natural tendency to put on weight while eating the same as your thin cousin—but you don't have to be fat; you can keep the weight off. You were meant to be thin and healthy. Don't let old excuses, old prejudices, or old friends cheat you of that.

ATTITUDE ADJUSTING

Before you began to lose weight, I explained to you that you would find dieting very difficult if you ate for all the wrong reasons. Have you licked those attitudes for good, or will you still find yourself running to food for comfort?

Perhaps the most demoralizing thing in the world is to overeat deliberately, knowing while you do it that you don't need the food and that it will make you fat. Binge . . . guilt . . . more binges . . .

more guilt. Once back on that downward spiral, you'll find it very hard to break out.

So I'm going to tell you one thing that you're probably not going to like very much, but it needs to be said: Your compulsive need to overeat is a symptom of discontent—worry, frustration, boredom, restriction, and so on. Food isn't the basic problem, and you must look beyond that in order to cure your weight problem for good.

You can do this in three stages.

First, find a substitute. It shouldn't be alcohol, drugs, or tobacco, of course. It could be a friend or neighbor, a parent, a child, a pen pal, a counselor. A cookie is no substitute for a good listener or some good advice.

Second, every single time you feel like turning to food as a substitute for any other aspect of life, get in the habit of doing something positive. A binge lowers your self-esteem and in the long run makes your problems seem worse. Positive action of almost any kind will raise your self-esteem, and you will be on an upward spiral instead. What is a positive action? Anything at all that gives pleasure, help, enjoyment, or enlightenment to you—or to anyone else. It could be anything from reading a book or magazine to visiting an elderly neighbor, to taking up a hobby, tidying up neglected cupboards, or joining an evening class. Do it once; you'll see I'm right. Do it several times; you're winning. From small positive actions, it's but a small step to stage three.

Third, set to work on those major areas of discontent in your life, or whatever it is about yourself that is really bugging you. Go on—don't accept your life as it is; really think about what's wrong. Don't be frightened of life and all it has to offer. You lost weight, so you can do anything. That should be your attitude. Don't be paralyzed by fear of failure. That was the old you. The new you works out what is wrong, what you can do about it, and if you think you can't do anything—why not?

All this will take more nerve and more effort than overeating does. But at the end of the day, food is only food.

Life is more than just a jelly doughnut.

And you, too, deserve your share.

A SUMMARY OF WHAT YOU'VE READ IN CHAPTER 10

- *Staying* thin is even more important than getting thin.
- You don't have to "eat like a rabbit" for the rest of your life in order to stay thin.
- You do have to eat a little less than you did when you were overweight.
- People's calorie needs vary widely; don't compare yourself with others.
- Gradually build up the amount of food you eat after dieting for a while until you discover your own maintenance level.
- Keep a regular eye on the scale to ensure you never gain more than a very few pounds.
- Accept food for what it is, and accept yourself as a thin person—for life!

✤ 11. ✤

Junk Food
for Kids

At dinnertime every day of the year throughout the country, millions of mothers serve beefburgers and fries or fish sticks and chips to their appreciative children—and feel deeply, uncontrollably guilty for doing so.

Kids love all the things that we've been led to believe are "bad" for them, and most would rather starve than eat brown rice, broccoli, or boiled fish. No wonder that even the most well-intentioned parents give up the fight to provide their children with a "healthier" diet. What all parents want is for their children to be healthy, strong, fit, and slim. But they also—very badly—want them to enjoy their food.

In this chapter, I aim to prove that the two ideas are compatible, and that many of your worries about your children's diet are unfounded.

CHILDREN'S NUTRITIONAL REQUIREMENTS*

Although there are broad similarities between what children need and what adults need for good health, there are also some important differences.

You'll have read in Chapter 2 (refresh your memory now!) about a good adult diet. Here are the main differences when it comes to your children:

- Children's protein needs in relation to their size are higher than an adult's (see Table 8, page 234). An average eleven-year-old boy needs more protein than most women; so does an eleven-year-old girl.
- Children of all ages need more calcium than adults, apart from women who are pregnant or breast-feeding. Their need for calcium is so high because they are forming bones and teeth. Need peaks at adolescence, when the recommended dietary allowance is 1,200 milligrams. To help convert the calcium to strong bone, children also need sufficient vitamin D. In summer enough is supplied by sunlight on skin, but in winter a daily 10 unigrams is recommended.
- Iron needs are high in relation to size. A six-year-old child needs as much iron as an adult male, and by the time she's eleven a girl needs more than a man (see Table 8, page 234).
- A high-fiber diet is not necessarily a good idea unless your child is constipated or tends toward being overweight. Because children's nutrient needs are high in relation to the size of their digestive systems and stomachs, a very high-bulk

---
* Age four and over.

TABLE 8

CHILDREN'S NUTRIENT NEEDS—DAILY*

Age	Calories	Protein (g)	Calcium (mg)	Iron (mg)	Vitamin C (mg)
Boys					
4–6	1,700	30	800	10	45
7–10	2,400	34	800	10	45
11–14	2,700	45	1200	18	50
15–18	2,800	56	1200	18	60
Comparison with an adult male 23–50, moderately active	2,700	56	800	10	60
Girls					
4–6	1,700	30	800	10	45
7–10	2,400	34	800	10	45
11–14	2,200	46	1200	18	50
15–18	2,200	46	1200	18	60
Comparison with an adult female 23–50, most occupations	2,000	44	800	18	60

*National Research Council, National Academy of Sciences Recommended Dietary Allowances, Ninth Edition Selection, 1980.

diet may mean they simply cannot eat enough to satisfy those requirements.

- And, last, children's calorie needs are high in relation to their size. By the time a boy is seven or eight, he may be needing more calories than his mother, for example (see Table 8 above). This means they need plenty of carbohydrate-rich foods to supply that energy.

Children also need all the other nutrients that adults need: enough vitamin C and all the other vitamins, minerals, and trace elements, in correspondingly smaller amounts.

How important is it to limit the amount of fat, sugar, and salt in your children's diet?

Although our taste in food usually changes as we grow older, the diet we eat as children plays a large part in deciding what we eat as adults. Although young children rarely suffer from the type of heart disease that adults get or have high blood pressure, and they certainly don't succumb to mid-life-onset diabetes, what your children eat at ten years old will give them habits that last a lifetime. So it is important that the habits learned are good ones. It's wise that they should learn to enjoy a diet that doesn't contain too much animal fat; that they should not get into the habit of eating too much high-salt food, or of adding salt to food at the table; and, for the sake of their future waistline and good health, as well as the immediate well-being of their teeth, that they should, perhaps most important of all, not develop an obsessive liking for very sweet, sugary foods.

So how does a "junk food" diet fit in with these rather exacting nutritional requirements? In many respects, quite well. In fact, parents who are over-enthusiastic in their attempts to give their children a healthy diet may be doing more harm than good.

Let's look again at children's special needs in the context of a "junk food" diet.

SPECIAL NUTRIENT NEEDS

Plenty of calories

The fact that some "junk food" can be fattening is of
relevance only if your child is putting on large
amounts of weight. But for most parents, the problem is more likely to be one of finding enough food
to give a ravenous child who never seems to put on
an ounce! The best way to supply your children with
calories is to give them "high-density" foods, meat
and cheese, bread, pasta. Fat is the highest-density
food there is, so you can include a sensible amount
of butter or margarine and properly fried foods in a
thin child's diet without feeling guilty. Many of the
so-called "junk" foods aimed specifically at kids—
fish sticks; burgers; hot dogs, grilled, broiled, or
baked—are not high in fat, and most children have
a natural aversion to eating fat that's been left on
cooked meat—roast beef or bacon, for instance. So
as long as you apply all the rules and guidelines
regarding fat that appeared in the adult Junk Food
Diet to your child's diet, too (limit fat to 30 percent
of total calories), you won't need to worry.

So don't feel guilty about those fries—a well-
cooked plateful supplies not only calories for a hungry growing child, but also some valuable vitamin
C, some protein, and carbohydrates. What you don't
want to do when your children are hungry is give
them a candy bar. Sweet foods will satisfy hunger
only for a short time; they contain no "goodness"
and will give the wrong idea about sensible eating.
More about sweet foods later, though.

Plenty of protein

Many "junk" foods are a good source of protein—all
of those based on lean beef, poultry, and fish are
good additions to your child's diet. Eggs, low-fat sausages, frankfurters, and low-fat cold cuts are good
protein sources. And most of the carbohydrate-rich
foods like potatoes and bread contain reasonable
amounts of protein. Some of these foods have a medium or high added-salt content, so if you're watching salt in your child's diet, it's worth limiting the
higher-salt items (see Table 9, page 238) to occasional meals, and make sure never to let your child
add salt to meals at the table.

Plenty of calcium

The best sources of calcium are milk (whole, low-fat,
and skim), yogurt, and hard cheeses, all of which
also provide other valuable nutrients, such as protein. Four cups of milk a day will give your children
their full day's calcium requirement. A container of
yogurt will provide one-third, as will enough cheese
for a sandwich.

Although cottage cheese and skim-milk soft
cheeses are much lower in fat than Cheddar, they
have a relatively low calcium content, so I think
that the higher-fat Cheddar, cheese spreads, and
medium-fat soft cheeses are a better bet for children. The only other foods with appreciable
amounts of calcium per serving are sardines (if your
child eats the bones, which many won't), and leafy
green vegetables.

So you begin to see why dairy products are so val-

TABLE 9

HIGH-SALT FOODS
(excluding reduced-salt versions, which will be clearly labeled)

bouillon cubes and concentrates	corned beef
brine-cured vegetables, such as sauerkraut and pickles	frankfurters
	ham
	sardines
canned tomato juice and vegetable juices	cheese sauce
	ketchup
breads, crackers, rolls, and snacks with salted tops	prepared mustard
	horseradish
	olives
potato chips with salt	pickles
peanuts with salt	canned soups
pretzels with salt	cheese
smoked fish	processed cheese
bacon	cold cuts

uable for children, especially ones who won't "eat their spinach."

If your children don't like plain milk or natural yogurt, it is far better to let them drink chocolate milk or a hot chocolate and eat fruit yogurt, or even custard, rice pudding, or ice cream than to see them go short of their calcium.

Plenty of iron

Your child may be one of the few children who adores liver and begs for it—but if he or she does, you're in the minority! Liver is the best source of iron, but next best are all the red meats. (That maligned beefburger is looking more like the good guy every minute, isn't it?) Eggs, peas, beans, and fortified breakfast cereals are also good sources of iron. Even chocolate contains some iron.

So is junk food absolved?

Children who eat cornflakes or Rice Krispies for breakfast, a burger and (properly cooked) fries for lunch at school, spaghetti when they get home, plus Cheddar cheese and crackers as a snack later are certainly not eating what I would call junk food—not by any means. As far as it goes, such a diet goes a long way toward providing them with all the nutrients they need for good health. But where your child's diet is likely to go wrong from here on in can occur in two important ways:

First, it may not get the addition of fruit and vegetables that your child needs for the vital vitamins and minerals they supply.

It is a very unusual child who isn't fussy about one vegetable or another. Highest on the hate-list is anything green and leafy—cabbage and brussels sprouts, for instance. But don't give up on all vegetables because children refuse one or two. Your children need vegetables and fruit, and there will always be something they are going to like—or at least eat without too much coaxing.

A fairly comprehensive list of the best sources of vitamin C appears on page 44.

Second, the addition of too many sweet and/or fatty and/or salty and/or low-nutrient snacks and extras may turn a perfectly healthy "junk food" diet into a less healthy one, if you aren't careful. Even worse, if you aren't careful, these low-nutrient snack foods may become so appealing to your children that they begin to replace the higher-quality foods in their diet.

Here are my guidelines on the subject for a child who is thin or within the normal weight range for his or her height (there are different guidelines for overweight children toward the end of the chapter):

- If your child has a big appetite, get into the habit of satisfying his or her hunger with a bread snack or nut and fruit snacks. If the diet is not otherwise very high in salt, there is nothing wrong with the occasional bag of potato chips; in fact, the new-style potato chips, cooked with the skin left on in oil with not too much added salt, are a nutritious snack and a reasonable addition to a lunchbox.
- If your child likes cakes and/or cookies, give him or her the lower-sugar varieties that do contain various nutrients—fruitcake or carrot cake, peanut butter or oatmeal cookies, for example, rather than sponge cake; or sugar-icing-coated cookies.
- Yogurts, custards, and all milk-based puddings are a better bet for a child than sherbet and ices, if you want to give your child a dessert. Fruit-based puddings are best of all.
- If your child asks for candy, limit it to a definite time—say, on weekends only, or a little after dinner.

- Most candy contains nothing but sugar, water, colorings, and flavorings, and add nothing whatsoever to the goodness of your child's diet. Chewy candies, jellies, gums, toffees, and any sweet, gooey, sticky foods are the ones that are most likely to leave the deposits on your child's teeth that start the process leading to tooth decay.

- Try to give sugary foods as part of a meal rather than on their own, and remember that the longer the sweet food is in contact with your child's teeth, the more potential damage it can do, so it is better to give a child a candy bar or any sweet item that he or she can eat right away rather than, say, a roll of hard candies that he or she may suck for hours.

- Get your child into the habit of cleaning his or her teeth after every meal and/or after every time he or she has eaten a sugary food. Since a child can't (or doesn't) clean his or her teeth at school, it is best not to include high-sugar items in your child's lunchbox.

- Don't replace nutritious drinks such as fruit juice and milk with low-nutrient or no-nutrient drinks like cola and soft drinks. Sugary drinks are similar to many candies in that they usually contain nothing but sugar, water, colorings, and flavorings—so use them only occasionally. The cheapest drink to quench thirst is water!

- Don't allow your child to eat candy, cookies, popcorn, and the like instead of a meal.

- If your child doesn't have a sweet tooth, don't encourage one to develop with regular bribes or presents of cookies and candy.

Limit—or ban?

The reason I say sweet foods and snacks should be limited in your children's diet rather than completely banned is simple: If there is one way to ensure that children want something, it is to tell them they can't have it. Add to that the natural fascination of something that is forbidden and you have children who will, once they're out of school age, find a supply of candy bars, chocolate, or whatever, despite your best efforts. That way you have no control.

However, if you offer your children a sensible compromise—the occasional item—they will be less concerned about it. In other words, those sweet treats and extras should be limited in your child's diet in just the same way they are on the adult Junk Food Diet and maintenance plan.

By doing this, you will be getting your children used to the idea of balance, variety, and moderation in their diet, an idea that will do them nothing but good all their life.

How do you know you're helping them to get the balance right? If they're not overweight, if they're in good health with a full set of teeth and go for regular dental checkups, you're doing okay.

Table 10

TRAFFIC LIGHT GUIDE TO KIDS' "JUNK" FOOD

GREEN FOR GO

Food type
Children's favorite meals:
beefburgers, fish sticks, chicken fingers, turkey, pizza, hot dogs, spaghetti.
Your attitude should be:
Don't feel guilty if your children enjoy these foods. If you add vegetables and/or fruit to the meal, they are fine. Follow the "fat guidelines" above.

Food type
French fries
Your attitude should be:
If properly cooked, they are a good source of carbohydrates, protein, and vitamin C. But don't forget alternatives, like baked potatoes, or even mashed potatoes now and then!

Food type
White bread
Your attitude should be:
This is an excellent choice for most children—it's often fortified with extra iron. For extra fiber, soft-grain white is the ideal choice.

YELLOW FOR CAUTION

Food type
Puddings and desserts
Your attitude should be:
Yogurts, milk puddings, ice cream, and custard
all supply calcium. Fruit with calcium-rich ac-
companiment is a good pudding for kids, but sun-
daes and other gooey desserts are best kept as
occasional happenings.

Food type
Snacks—potato chips, salted peanuts
Your attitude should be:
They're fine in reasonable quantities for the hun-
gry child, but think about the salt content; choose
low-salt versions if possible.

Food type
Cake and cookies
Your attitude should be:
Think of them as occasional items.

RED FOR STOP

Food type
Candy and soft drinks
Your attitude should be:
These are high-sugar, low-nutrient foods. Limit
them severely.

JUNK FOOD AND ALLERGIES

Because additive-bashing is the current national pastime, it's little wonder that more and more parents are asking "Is it the additives?" when their child has a rash, is sick, has a runny nose, is lethargic or hyperactive (surely the most overused word of the decade).

The additives debate is never more fierce than when it concerns our kids. Let me say right now that no one is arguing the fact that some children are allergic to some additives. The most common food additives to cause a reaction in recent years have been yellow and red food dyes. However, nowadays it's hard to find foods that contain them—manufacturers wisely decided to find alternatives—but it is the food-dye group as a whole that appears to cause the most frequent problems.

Ironically, it is by no means the case that food additives are the biggest cause of allergic reactions —far from it. The items that most commonly trigger allergic reactions are wheat, milk, eggs, shellfish, strawberries, and nuts—all foods that we regard as "healthy" and "natural."

It is estimated that up to 25 percent of the population may have allergies, and that half of those allergies are food-related. The most common symptoms are tingling or itchy skin, rash, asthma, nausea, and diarrhea.

If you think your child may be allergic to a food or a food additive, talk to your doctor, who may suggest an elimination program to confirm the allergy, or other suitable treatment.

Don't forget that all additives in food on sale for human consumption in this country have been approved by the government after what it considers to be adequate testing. However, if you are one of the many parents who still prefer to cut down on additives "to be on the safe side," it is becoming an easier and easier task to do so.

First, the manufacturers are voluntarily removing many unnecessary additives from their products, especially artificial colorings (those dyes that cause most of the allergy problems that do occur) and flavorings that are really only in the foods for cosmetic purposes. And, second, because by law the manufacturer has to include a list of ingredients including additives on the packaging of all foods, it is a fairly easy matter to check the labels at the supermarket for the additives you want to avoid. This is particularly useful if there is just one you need to cut out.

OVERWEIGHT CHILDREN

Is your child overweight? Let's find out.

The height/weight graphs that follow (Tables 11–14, pages 253–256) will give you a fair guide to what your child's weight should be, but before you look at them, bear in mind the following:

- The heights and weights given for the ages are average for that age. The 50th percentile represents the average for a child of a particular age. It is important to consider both the height and weight graphs. If your child is at the 95th percentile for weight, and only at the 25th percentile for his or her age, then he or she is overweight. If, however, your child is at the 75th percentile for

both height and weight, he or she is probably at
the appropriate weight for his or her height.

- Remember that two children of the same age will
  vary in height and weight and still both be within
  an acceptable range.
- Use the charts in conjunction with your own common sense. For instance, do your children look
  overweight? Are they much heavier than all the
  other children in their class? How do they look
  without clothes on? Are they flabby? Do you find
  it hard to get clothes to fit them? For example,
  are the clothes at the right length but always too
  tight? You can probably tell more by using these
  visual methods than by using the graphs, which
  are only guides. Use the preceding points to help
  you make a sensible decision.

If you have come to the conclusion that, yes, your
child is overweight, what should you do?

Don't impose a very strict diet. Rather than put
him or her on an active weight-loss diet, it is probably better to put him or her on a "containing" diet
—one that will keep him or her at the same weight
for the next few months so that eventually he or she
will gain enough height to slim down naturally.
Most children grow an average of 2 to 3 inches a
year, which should result, depending upon his or
her age, in a surplus of about 5 pounds being "lost"
in this way.

What you don't want to do is totally ignore the
child's weight problem and hope that it will disappear of its own accord, without your having to keep
any kind of eye on what the child eats. Your child
needs your help and support in order to slim down.

Overeating, in childhood as in adulthood, is a habit that can be hard to break.

GETTING THE WEIGHT OFF

I am not going to give you a set low-calorie diet for your child, because calorie-counting depends so much on age, height, and a scale of problem and other factors. Also, if children are put "on a diet" and know it, they are more likely to rebel, or cheat, or get bored.

If you decide to devise your own diet, I'd strongly advise you *not* to put him or her on one that is less than 500 calories a day below the average calorie requirement for a child of that sex and age (see Table 8 on page 234)—and never for a child less than ten years old, unless directed to do so by your doctor. I would also advise that any weight loss above half a pound a week for a child is too high. It would make sense for you to consult a doctor if you think your child is seriously overweight.

So how do you achieve that weight loss without a diet as such?

This is what you do. Go back to the Traffic Light Guide to Kids' "Junk" Food (see Table 10, pages 243–244).

First, you cut back on all the Red foods in your child's diet—the sugary things that aren't giving any of the nutrients needed for health. If there has been a lot of this kind of item, you may have to cut back gradually, and replace some of them with more nutritious foods—trade a bag of chips for a bag of pretzels, for instance. You could also swap sugary colas and drinks for the calorie-free kind made with artificial sweeteners, although in the

long term it's best to get your child used to water or
fruit juice as a drink.

At the same time, you can swap whole milk for
skim milk, and butter in sandwiches, and so on, for
a low-fat spread. These are changes that will probably not even be noticed.

After a couple of weeks on this plan, weigh your
child. If any weight has been lost—say, a pound or
two—that could be enough on its own. If no weight
has been lost—perhaps because there weren't many
sweets in the diet anyway—move on to the next
step.

This is to replace the Yellow items on the chart
with lower-calorie ones, or to cut them out altogether. For example, you could replace a large slice
of chocolate cake with a small slice of sponge cake,
or three chocolate cookies with two plain ones. You
could replace a fruit pie and chocolate pudding with
low-fat fruit yogurt. Whatever you do, don't apolo-
gize when you hand over any of these trades. If you
don't mention the reason, the child will never get a
chance to feel deprived.

Get the scale out again in a couple of weeks. If a
pound or two has been lost, continue on the same
plan. I expect most children will be losing a little
weight by this time. If not, or if the weight loss is
marginal, proceed as follows.

Substitute all cake, cookies, and puddings for
fresh-fruit desserts or diet yogurts—but allow one
small treat a day, maximum of 150 calories. Cut
down on the amount of fries or trade them most of
the time with boiled potato or baked potato, and if
your child's been having large portions of his or her
main meal for his or her age, cut down on the
amount of food on the plate. You won't save all that

many calories by cutting down on the amount of vegetables (apart from fried ones), and in any case they help to fill the child up, so I'd cut down a little on meat, pastry, and cheese. Make sure gravy is skimmed of fat.

Don't cut down on fruit, and I wouldn't suggest cutting down drastically on bread, or plain rice or pasta, unless your child has literally been getting through half a loaf or potful or more a day.

Speaking of which, some children will be overweight because of an obsessive liking for one particular food—french fries, say, or cake or cookies, perhaps. Do all you can to get them to cut down on that food. If it's something they eat mostly at home, simply buy less. While freeing them of their obsession for this particular food, don't let them go hungry. Substitute other foods, especially low-calorie ones. Then, when you have the single-food fetish licked, you can begin the weight-loss process, using the method outlined above.

It is very hard to slim down a rebellious child, and for that reason it is essential that you keep his or her cooperation all along the line. With most children, this means doing it in the way I've described —getting them to lose weight without there ever being a point at which you say "You're going to diet." To this end, it will help a great deal if all the family make some, or all, of the diet changes I've outlined; if you've been following The Junk Food Diet yourself, you are probably halfway there already.

PLANNING YOUR CHILD'S MENU

Build up a healthy diet for your child with the help of the meal ideas and tips that follow.

No busy parent has the time to be a nutritionist. A large part of planning a good diet is instinctive. The most important rule, perhaps, is to vary your family's meals so that they don't have the same food too often (the exception, of course, being staples such as bread and potatoes, which can be eaten every day, and without which we would find providing meals very hard). A fairly simple way of ensuring that your child gets all the nutrients necessary for good health is to follow the Basic Four principle:

1. Give two servings a day from the Milk group, the foods rich in calcium. These are milk and milk products, such as yogurt.
2. Give four servings a day or more from the Bread and Cereal group, the foods rich in carbohydrates. These are potatoes, bread, rice, pasta, and breakfast cereals.
3. Give two servings a day from the Meat group. These are beef, pork, lamb, poultry, fish, eggs, and meat substitutes such as beans and legumes.
4. Give four servings a day or more of the Fruits and Vegetables group.

This plan oversimplifies food, because most of the foods overlap into other groups: for example, the Milk group also contains protein, the Meat-group foods are good sources of protein, and all the foods mentioned, not just fruits and vegetables, contain vitamins and minerals. However, it is a very good guideline to follow.

Another simple way to ensure reasonable nutrition is to make sure that at every meal your child has a protein-rich food, a carbohydrate-rich food, and a fruit or vegetable, plus a pint of milk a day.

A meal doesn't have to be a traditional "meat-and-potato-plus-vegetable" to be nutritious: You could get the right mix from a plate of beans (protein) on rice (carbohydrate), plus a piece of fresh fruit.

And the meal doesn't have to be cooked, either. A cold sandwich can be just as nutritious as a hot meal.

Here are some more tips that will help you plan your children's daily menu:

- Give them a breakfast every day. You may not eat, or need, breakfast, but a breakfast will ensure that your children get a percentage of the nutrients they need, and they may not get another chance to eat until lunchtime, which isn't a good idea. The alternative is that they will feel ravenous by morning-break time and, more than likely, will eat a sugary snack instead of something more nutritious.
- Give them a packed lunch, if possible, so that you can have control over what they eat. The second-best idea is for them to buy a school meal—even if there is a choice, most of the alternatives will be reasonably high in nutrients. The worst option is for your children to go outside the school and buy what they like. Research shows that they are then most likely to get a very unbalanced meal—a bag of chips, for instance, or even nothing at all.
- Remember, variety and balance are the key. The wider your choice of foods, the more likely your children are to get all they need for health.

Table 11

BOYS' HEIGHT: 2 to 18 Years Physical Growth NCHS* Percentiles

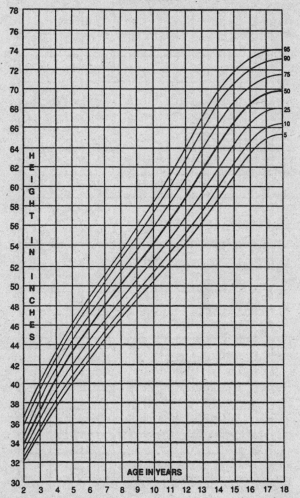

* National Center of Health Statistics.

Table 12

BOYS' WEIGHT: 2 to 18 Years Physical Growth NCHS* Percentiles

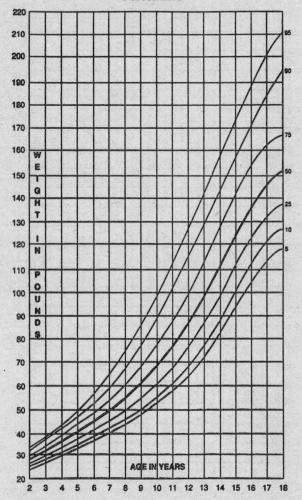

---

* National Center of Health Statistics.

Table 13

GIRLS' HEIGHT: 2 to 18 Years Physical Growth NCHS* Percentiles

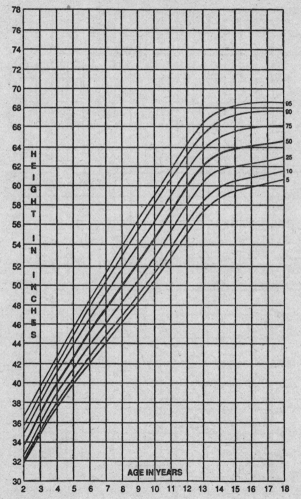

* National Center of Health Statistics.

Table 14

GIRLS' WEIGHT: 2 to 18 Years Physical Growth
NCHS* Percentiles

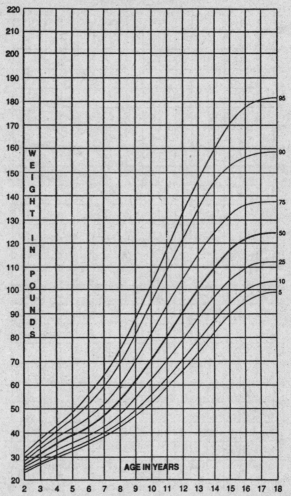

* National Center of Health Statistics.

✤ 12. ✤

The Junk Food Diet Recipes

You don't need to be a brilliant cook, or even an experienced one, to whip up the simple recipes that follow. And you certainly don't need a lot of spare time. So, although you can follow The Junk Food Diet perfectly well without using even one of these dishes, it's well worth giving some of them a try. They will add even more variety to your diet and are an added precaution against boredom!

Each recipe had to pass a very stringent test before I allowed it to be included! It had to fulfill at least six out of seven of the following criteria:

1. Easy to shop for, prepare, and cook.
2. Quick to prepare and cook. A few recipes have a long cooking time, but you can be doing something else while the cooking's in progress, so that isn't necessarily a negative point.
3. The bland and the dull have been banished. I know what your taste buds like.
4. Not depressingly obvious "diet dinners." I love meals that sound fattening when in fact they're not! And I don't see the point of cooking depressing-sounding dishes like "Dieter's Fish and Cel-

ery Casserole." I thought you would agree with me, which is why my recipes include such glorious meals as Chili Con Carne, Lasagna Rolls, Spaghetti with Meat Sauce, Fettuccine with Ham, and Beef Enchiladas!

5. Suitable for everyone. The recipes serve four, two, or one, depending upon which is most suitable for that particular dish. However, many of the family meals can quite easily be cooked in smaller quantities. Just divide the ingredients accordingly.

6. No hard-to-find ingredients or unfamiliar ones. Most of us are familiar with tortillas and sour cream by now, and that's about as "exotic" as you'll need to get.

7. Inexpensive. I've tried hard not to feature lobster, specialty produce, or smoked salmon. Most of the meals will fit in well with your food budget. One or two are more special, included deliberately in the hope that you'll want a celebration meal now and then—celebrating your weight loss, I expect.

The recipes can be used in two ways:

1. As part of your Junk Food Diet, in which case you'll find the number of the page(s) where the recipe appears at the top of each recipe. Calories given are per portion for the recipe only. Any suggested accompaniments or any foods that may accompany the dish within the diets are not included, which is why, for instance, a 400-calorie recipe may be included in the 500-calorie meal lists in the Pick Your Own Plan.

2. You can also use the recipes on your maintenance plan (see Chapter 10), as and when you wish.

Remember, with all recipes it is best to use the freshest ingredients you can find, and you should weigh or measure ingredients carefully.

Sauces

Cheese Sauce (see pages 119, 135, 146, 179, 278, 285)

Serves 4
Calories per portion: 160
Preparation and cooking time: 10 minutes

1 tablespoon butter or margarine
1 tablespoon flour
2 cups skim milk
4 ounces reduced-fat Cheddar-style cheese,
shredded
pinch salt and pepper

Melt butter or margarine in saucepan over medium heat. Gradually add flour and continue cooking for 1 minute, stirring constantly. Gradually add milk, stirring to avoid lumps. Add cheese and stir until blended. Add salt and pepper to taste.
NOTE: Make Parsley Sauce, at only 90 calories a portion, by omitting the cheese and adding instead 2 tablespoons of chopped fresh parsley.

Tomato Sauce (see pages 269, 270, 286)

Serves 4
Calories per portion: 90
Preparation and cooking time: 20 minutes

2 tablespoons olive or corn oil
1 medium onion, very finely chopped
1 15-ounce can tomatoes, chopped with their liquid
1 tablespoon tomato paste
2 garlic cloves, minced (optional)
1 teaspoon dried oregano or parsley

Heat oil in medium non-stick saucepan over medium heat. Add onion and cook over medium heat until transparent and soft. Add remainder of ingredients and simmer for about 15 minutes, until a thick sauce forms. This should have enough salt, but you can add a little if you must! For a smoother sauce, put through blender.

Barbecue Sauce (see pages 134, 145, 276)

Serves 4
Calories per portion: 60
Preparation and cooking time: 10 minutes

1 tablespoon olive or corn oil
1 tablespoon red-wine vinegar
1 tablespoon honey
1 heaping tablespoon tomato paste
2 tablespoons soy sauce
1 envelope instant beef broth
1 teaspoon mixed herbs
pinch cayenne pepper
4 tablespoons water
1 garlic clove, minced

Blend all ingredients thoroughly in a bowl. Then
bring to boil in small saucepan and simmer for a
few minutes until there is a rich, coating sauce.
(Even if you think you don't like garlic, do try the
garlic in this recipe!)

BREAD SNACKS

Pizza Toasts (see pages 131, 142, 166, 168)

Serves 2
Calories per portion: 300
Preparation and cooking time: 10 minutes

2 large slices bread (from a round loaf, if possible)
1 small onion, finely chopped
1 8-ounce can tomatoes, drained and chopped
¼ cup mushrooms, sliced, or red pepper
4 ounces reduced-fat Cheddar-style cheese, grated
dried oregano

Toast bread. Mix together onion, tomatoes, and mushrooms. Spread half the cheese on the bread, followed by tomato mixture, then remainder of cheese. Pop under broiler until cheese is melted and golden.

Tuna Pita (see pages 164, 168)

Serves 2
Calories per serving: 400
Preparation time: 5 minutes

2 small pita pockets
1 6½-ounce can tuna, drained
2 tomatoes, roughly chopped
4 scallions, chopped
1-inch cucumber, chopped
2 tablespoons reduced-calorie mayonnaise

Warm pitas (optional). Mix together all other ingredients and divide between split and opened pita pockets.

Egg and Cheese Meals

Spanish Scramble (see pages 161, 166, 172)

Serves 2
Calories per portion: 230
Preparation and cooking time: 10 minutes

1 tablespoon butter or margarine
1 medium onion, finely chopped
1/4 cut green and/or red pepper, sliced
2 fresh tomatoes, or 2 well-drained canned
ones, chopped
3 medium eggs
2 tablespoons skim milk
pinch salt and pepper

Melt butter or margarine in non-stick frying pan
and stir-fry vegetables for a few minutes until soft.
Beat eggs, milk, and seasonings in a bowl and pour
into pan. Cook over low heat, stirring, until eggs are
scrambled.

Potato Frittata (see pages 128, 140)

Serves 2
Calories per portion: 235
Preparation and cooking time: 10 minutes

1 tablespoon butter or margarine
2 teaspoons corn oil
1 medium onion, thinly sliced
2 small potatoes, boiled and sliced
3 medium eggs
2 tablespoons skim milk
salt and pepper to taste
few chopped chives or scallions, fresh or dried

Melt butter and oil in non-stick frying pan and fry onion and potatoes until golden. Beat eggs with milk, seasoning, and chives and pour over vegetables in pan. Cook over medium heat until eggs are set. If you like, you can brown the frittata under a broiler. Cut frittata in half, slide it carefully from pan, and serve.

FISH MEALS

Tuna Florentine (see pages 125, 135, 147, 174)

Serves 4
Calories per portion: 300
Preparation and cooking time: 40 minutes

1 15-ounce can tomatoes, drained and chopped
1 tablespoon tomato paste
2 tablespoons flour
2 cups mushrooms, sliced
1 garlic clove, minced
1 teaspoon Italian seasoning
pinch salt if necessary
2 6½-to-7-ounce cans tuna in water, well
drained
½ 10-ounce package frozen chopped spinach,
thawed
1 cup plain non-fat yogurt
2 teaspoons cornstarch
3 ounces reduced-fat Cheddar-style cheese,
shredded

In a bowl, mix together tomatoes, tomato paste,
flour, mushrooms, garlic, seasoning, and tuna (in
fairly large chunks). Spoon into a 4-cup ovenproof
dish. Spread spinach over the top. Mix together yogurt, cornstarch, most of the cheese, and salt (if you
wish to), and spread over top. Sprinkle on remainder of cheese. Bake at 325° F. until top is golden and
casserole is heated through, about 25 minutes.

Fisherman's Soup (see pages 119, 171, 172)

Serves 4
Calories per serving 200
Preparation and cooking time: 45 minutes

1 tablespoon olive oil
1 cup onion, chopped
1 garlic clove, minced
1 14-ounce can stewed tomatoes, with liquid
2 tablespoons tomato paste
1 bay leaf
2 cups water
1/4 cup chopped cilantro or parsley
1/2 cup dry white wine
1 8-ounce bottle clam juice
1 16-ounce package frozen codfish fillets, partially defrosted
2 to 3 dashes hot pepper sauce (optional)
lemon slices

In large saucepan, sauté onion and garlic in olive oil until onion is transparent, about 10 minutes. Add tomatoes and their liquid, tomato paste, bay leaf, water, and cilantro. Simmer, covered, for 15 minutes. Add wine, clam juice, and codfish. Simmer, covered, an additional 15 minutes. Stir in hot pepper sauce. Serve with lemon slices and additional chopped cilantro, if desired.

Shrimp Provençale (see pages 123, 170)

Serves 4
Calories per portion: 155
Preparation and cooking time: 15 minutes

1 tablespoon butter or margarine
1 small onion, finely chopped
1 garlic clove, minced
3/4 cup mushrooms, sliced
1 tablespoon all-purpose flour
1/2 cup dry white wine, or equivalent amount
of cooking wine
1 6-ounce bottle clam juice or water
salt and pepper to taste
1 tablespoon tomato paste
1 8-ounce can tomatoes, chopped
3/4 pound cleaned shrimp, fresh or frozen

Melt butter or margarine in frying pan and cook
onion over medium heat until transparent and soft.
Add garlic and mushrooms and cook 2 minutes
more. Add flour and stir to blend. Add wine. Allow
to bubble for a minute. Then add clam juice, seasoning, tomato paste, chopped tomatoes, and shrimp.
Simmer for a few minutes or until shrimp curl and
turn pink.

Cod Creole (see pages 125, 172)

Serves 4
Calories per portion: 250
Preparation and cooking time: 55 minutes

Tomato Sauce for 4 (see recipe, page 260)
1¼ pounds codfish fillets, cut into four pieces,
or 4 5-ounce fish steaks
2 teaspoons brown sugar
little Tabasco, or ½ teaspoon chili seasoning
2 teaspoons Worcestershire sauce
1 small green pepper, chopped

Make tomato sauce and keep warm. Place codfish in a shallow ovenproof baking dish. Mix sugar, Tabasco, and Worcestershire sauce into tomato sauce and pour over the codfish. Sprinkle the chopped pepper on the mixture. Cover and cook at 300° F. for 30 minutes, or until fish flakes when tested with a fork.

Fish Kebabs (see pages 130, 141, 162, 173)

Serves 4
Calories per portion: 300
Preparation and cooking time: 30 minutes

1/2 **quantity of Tomato Sauce (see recipe, page
260)**
2 **tablespoons honey**
2 **tablespoons soy sauce**
1 **teaspoon prepared mustard**
1 **pound fish fillets, cubed (such as monkfish,
swordfish, tuna, or halibut)**
4 **slices bacon, cut into squares**
1 **small red pepper, cut into squares**
1 **small green pepper, cut into squares**
12 **button mushrooms**
2 **teaspoons corn oil**

Make tomato sauce (you could make a full quantity
and freeze the remaining half) and add to it the
honey, soy sauce, and mustard. Thread fish, bacon,
and vegetables onto four long kebab sticks and
brush with oil. Broil under medium heat (or barbecue) for 10 to 12 minutes. Serve with the hot sauce.

POULTRY

Chicken Supreme

Serves 4
Calories per portion: 250
Preparation and cooking time: 40 minutes

4 chicken breast halves, boned and skinned
salt and pepper
2 tablespoons dry or medium-dry sherry, or
lemon juice
3/4 cup chicken broth
1 1/2 cups mushrooms, sliced
2 tablespoons low-fat margarine
1 tablespoon all-purpose flour
3/4 cup skim milk
1/4 cup light cream
4 sprigs parsley for garnish

Rub chicken with salt and pepper and put into shallow baking dish. Add sherry, chicken broth, and mushrooms and bring to a boil. Simmer gently for 25 minutes. With slotted spatula remove chicken and keep warm. Melt margarine in a saucepan and add flour. Cook for 1 or 2 minutes. Mix broth with milk and gradually add to the saucepan to make a sauce, stirring all the time. Stir in cream. Check seasoning, and pour over chicken. Garnish with parsley. (Lemon juice instead of sherry will yield an equally nice dish.)

Tandoori Chicken (see pages 120, 164, 171)

Serves 4
Calories per serving: 200
Preparation and cooking time: 45 minutes
Marinating time: 8 hours

2 whole chicken breasts, skinned and split
2 garlic cloves
1-inch piece fresh ginger, peeled
1 teaspoon chili powder
1/2 teaspoon salt
1 teaspoon curry powder
1/4 teaspoon ground cumin
1/4 teaspoon ground cinnamon
1/4 teaspoon ground cloves
1 cup plain non-fat yogurt
2 teaspoons fresh lemon juice

Cut 2 slits in each piece of chicken. Place chicken in plastic sealable bag. In a food processor with knife blade attached or in blender grind the garlic, ginger, chili powder, salt, curry powder, cumin, cinnamon, and cloves into a paste. Combine with yogurt and lemon juice. Pour over chicken in bag; seal. Refrigerate 8 hours, or overnight. Heat oven to 325° F. Remove chicken from bag and place in baking dish. Bake for 30 to 45 minutes, or until fork-tender, turning once.

Turkey Meat Loaf (see pages 123, 127, 133, 144)

Serves 6
Calories per serving: 300
Preparation and cooking time: 1 hour and 15
minutes

2 pounds turkey, ground
1 medium sweet red pepper, chopped
1 medium sweet green pepper, chopped
¼ cup celery, chopped
1 small onion, chopped
1 egg, beaten
2 teaspoons poultry seasoning
2 thin slices white or whole-wheat bread,
crumbled
1 tablespoon Dijon-style mustard
1 teaspoon water

Spray 13-×-9-inch baking dish with vegetable cooking spray. In large bowl, combine turkey, red pepper, green pepper, celery, onion, egg, poultry
seasoning, and bread. Blend all ingredients well. In
greased baking dish, shape into meat loaf. Combine
mustard and water and spread over meat loaf. Bake
at 350° F for 50 to 60 minutes, or until meat ther-
mometer inserted into loaf registers 185° F.

Chicken and Broccoli Casserole (see pages 120, 161, 171)

Serves 4
Calories per serving: 220
Preparation and cooking time: 25 minutes

2 whole chicken breasts, skinned, boned, and split
1 cup chicken broth
1 tablespoon cornstarch
2 tablespoons lemon juice
1/4 teaspoon salt
1 10-ounce package frozen broccoli spears, thawed
2 slices reduced-fat Cheddar-style cheese

In large skillet sprayed with vegetable cooking spray, brown chicken over medium heat. Remove chicken. Combine chicken broth, cornstarch, lemon juice, and salt. Stir into skillet and deglaze at high heat, scraping any browned bits from bottom of pan. Return chicken to skillet and arrange broccoli on top. Cover and cook 10 minutes, or until chicken is fork-tender. Top with cheese slices. Remove from heat and let stand, covered, 1 minute, or until cheese melts.

Chicken Curry (see pages 131, 142, 164, 173, 175)

Serves 4
Calories per portion: 315
Preparation and cooking time: 35 minutes

1 tablespoon corn oil
1 large onion, chopped
1 tablespoon curry powder (or to taste)
1 pound leftover cooked chicken meat
1 tablespoon flour
1 garlic clove, minced
1/2 cup raisins
chicken broth
1 tablespoon tomato paste
1 apple, sliced
1/2 cup non-fat plain yogurt
salt and pepper

Heat oil in a frying pan and cook onion until soft and just turning golden. Add curry powder and cook, stirring, for 1 or 2 minutes. Toss chicken in flour, then add to pan and cook for 2 more minutes. Add garlic and raisins, then the broth mixed with the tomato paste. Finally, add the apple, and simmer for 25 minutes. Stir yogurt in before serving. Taste and season with salt and pepper.

Turkey Kebabs (see pages 170, 173)

Serves 4
Calories per portion: 200
Preparation and cooking time: 25 minutes
Marinating time: up to 2 hours

1 quantity Barbecue Sauce (see recipe, page 261)
12 ounces fresh turkey breast
4 low-fat breakfast sausage links
1 small onion, quartered and split
1 medium zucchini, sliced
1 medium sweet red pepper, cut into squares

Make barbecue sauce and keep warm. Cut turkey and sausage into bite-sized pieces and thread alternately onto metal skewers with onion, zucchini, and pepper. If time permits, marinate kebabs in sauce for up to 2 hours; if not, it doesn't matter. Broil or barbecue kebabs under medium heat, basting with a little of the sauce from time to time.

Paradise Chicken (see pages 160, 173)

Serves 4
Calories per portion: 340
Preparation and cooking time: 10 minutes

1 pound cooked chicken or turkey meat, diced
1/4 cup white wine, or 2 tablespoons lemon
juice
6 tablespoons reduced-calorie mayonnaise
1 tablespoon mild curry powder
1 tablespoon apricot jam
8-ounce container plain non-fat yogurt
1 teaspoon onion powder
2 tablespoons raisins
1/2 cup chopped celery or apple (optional)

Blend all ingredients together well and chill before
serving.

PASTA AND RICE

Macaroni and Cheese (see pages 117, 173)

Serves 4
Calories per portion: 370
Preparation and cooking time: 30 minutes

**6 ounces uncooked macaroni
1 quantity cheese sauce (see recipe page 259)
pinch of nutmeg
2 tomatoes
2 ounces reduced-fat cheddar-style cheese,
shredded**

Cook the macaroni in a large pan of boiling, lightly salted water until just tender or as label directs. Drain. Meanwhile, make the cheese sauce. Pour the drained macaroni and the sauce into an ovenproof dish with the nutmeg. Slice the tomatoes and arrange them nicely over the top of the macaroni cheese. Top with the grated cheese and bake uncovered at 350° F. for 20 minutes, or until top is golden.

Fettuccine with Ham (see pages 133, 144, 175)

Serves 2
Calories per portion: 475
Preparation and cooking time: 15 minutes

4 ounces uncooked fettuccine (half-white, half-green is best)
1/2 10-ounce package frozen peas
1 cup button mushrooms, sliced
1/2 cup chicken broth
1/4 pound boiled ham, diced
pinch of mixed herbs
pinch pepper and salt, if necessary
1/3 cup light cream
1 tablespoon Parmesan cheese

Cook fettuccine in large pot of boiling water until just tender, or as label directs. Drain. Meanwhile, cook peas and mushrooms in broth in frying pan, then add ham to heat through. Add herbs and pepper. Add cream to frying pan, toss with pasta, and warm through. Check seasoning and serve on pasta with cheese sprinkled over.

Pasta Shells with Tuna (see page 176)

Serves 2
Calories per portion: 500
Preparation and cooking time: 15 minutes

3 ounces pasta shells, uncooked
1/2 cup plain non-fat yogurt
4 tablespoons reduced-calorie mayonnaise
2 tablespoons lemon juice
1 tablespoon parsley, chopped
salt and pepper
1 61/2- to-7-ounce can tuna in water, drained
and flaked
2 medium eggs, hard-cooked and chopped

Cook pasta shells in pot of boiling water until just tender, or as label directs. Drain and leave to cool. Mix together the yogurt, mayonnaise, lemon juice, parsley, and seasoning, and add tuna, eggs, and pasta. Toss and serve.
NOTE: A teaspoon of curry powder added to this dish makes a nice change and adds no extra calories.

Spaghetti with Meat Sauce (see page 176)

Serves 4
Calories per portion: 565
Preparation and cooking time: 30 minutes

1 quantity Basic Beef (see recipe, page 284)
1 8-ounce can tomatoes with liquid, chopped
2 garlic cloves, minced
8 ounces uncooked spaghetti
2 tablespoons Parmesan cheese

Cook basic beef and add tomatoes and garlic. Heat to boiling. Reduce heat to low; partially cover and simmer 20 minutes, or until thick, stirring regularly. Toward the end of cooking time, boil spaghetti in a large pot of lightly salted water until just tender, or as label directs. Drain and serve, topped with sauce and cheese.

Vegetable Lasagna Rolls (see pages 20, 129, 140, 163, 173)

Serves 4
Calories per serving: 350
Preparation and cooking time: 60 minutes

8 lasagna noodles
1 cup low-fat ricotta cheese
1 10-ounce package frozen spinach, chopped, thawed
1/2 cup shredded carrots
1 egg, beaten
1/4 teaspoon salt
1 8-ounce can tomato sauce
1/2 teaspoon garlic powder
1 teaspoon basil, dried
1/2 cup shredded part-skim mozzarella
2 tablespoons Parmesan cheese, grated

Cook noodles according to package directions. Drain. Rinse and drain again. Set aside. Spray a 9-×-9-inch baking dish with vegetable cooking spray. In small bowl combine ricotta, spinach, carrots, egg, and salt. Spread 2 tablespoons of filling over a noodle and roll it up. Place it standing up in baking dish. Repeat with remaining noodles and filling. In another small bowl, combine tomato sauce with garlic and basil. Spoon over rolled lasagna, sprinkle with cheeses, and cover with foil. Bake at 350° F. for 35 minutes. Uncover and bake 5 minutes more.

Risotto (see pages 123, 164, 173)

Serves 4
Calories per portion: 315
Preparation and cooking time: 1 hour

1 tablespoon low-fat margarine
1 cup long-grain rice
1 cup chicken meat, diced
1 medium onion, finely chopped
1 garlic clove, minced
3 1/2 cups chicken broth
1 tablespoon lemon juice
1 teaspoon turmeric powder, or saffron
salt and pepper to taste
1/2 10-ounce package frozen peas
lemon wedges for garnish

Melt low-fat margarine in large non-stick frying
pan. Add rice and stir to coat. Stir-fry for 1 or 2
minutes. Add remainder of ingredients, except peas.
Heat to boiling, reduce heat to low, and simmer for
35 minutes, uncovered, stirring occasionally. Add
peas and cook for 5 minutes more. Serve garnished
with lemon wedges.
NOTE: Should risotto get too dry, add a little more
broth during cooking.

RED MEAT DISHES

Basic Beef (see pages 281, 285)

Serves 6
Calories per portion: 220
Preparation and cooking time: 30 minutes

1 large onion, finely chopped
1 pound ground beef, very lean
1 stalk celery, chopped
1 large carrot, finely chopped
1 tablespoon tomato paste
1 teaspoon mixed herbs
1 cup beef broth
1 teaspoon Worcestershire sauce
salt and pepper to taste

Cook onion and beef in non-stick frying pan over medium heat until onion is soft and transparent. Stir to break up meat. Add vegetables and stir. Add remainder of ingredients and simmer for 20 minutes, or until beef is cooked through. Carefully spoon off any fat on top and discard (though, if the beef is very lean, there shouldn't be much).
NOTE: You can freeze this dish in full, half, or quarter portions for future use.

Moussaka (see pages 136, 147, 175, 176)

Serves 4
Calories per portion: 430
Preparation and cooking time: 1 hour 15 minutes

1 large or 2 small eggplants, about 1 pound
1 quantity Basic Beef (see recipe, page 284)
15-ounce can tomatoes, drained and chopped
1/2 quantity Cheese Sauce (see recipe, page 259)
2 ounces reduced-fat Cheddar-style cheese, shredded

Cut eggplant into 1/2-inch slices (don't peel it) and blanch in boiling water for 5 minutes. Drain and pat dry. Meanwhile, make basic beef and add tomatoes, and make cheese sauce. In an ovenproof baking dish, put beef, followed by eggplant slices, and top with sauce. Sprinkle shredded cheese on top and bake at 375° F. for 45 minutes, or until top is golden and bubbling.

Chili Con Carne (see pages 116, 133, 144, 164, 172)

Serves 4
Calories per serving: 330
Preparation and cooking time: 45 minutes

1 quantity Basic Beef (see recipe, page 284)
1 15-ounce can red kidney beans, drained
1 green pepper, finely chopped
1 teaspoon chili powder (or to taste)

Make basic beef. Add beans, pepper, and chili powder. Simmer for 20 minutes or longer.

Beef Enchiladas (see pages 136, 139, 147, 175, 176)

Serves 4
Calories per portion: 440
Preparation and cooking time: 30 minutes

1 8-ounce can corned beef
1 8-ounce can red kidney beans, drained
1 quantity Tomato Sauce (see recipe, page 260)
pinch chili powder
8 corn tortillas
1 tablespoon Parmesan cheese

Mash corned beef and kidney beans in a bowl, together with one-third of tomato sauce, and add chili powder. Fill each tortilla with a heaping spoonful of mixture, roll up, and place in a shallow ovenproof baking dish. Pour remainder of tomato sauce over tortillas and bake at 300° F. for 20 minutes, or until well heated through. Sprinkle with cheese and serve.

Beef Goulash (see pages 118, 124, 128, 162, 173)

Serves 4
Calories per portion: 300
Preparation and cooking time: 2 hours

2 tablespoons flour
1 tablespoon paprika
1 pound lean, trimmed stewing beef, cubed
1 tablespoon corn oil
1 large green pepper, sliced
1 large onion, sliced
1 cup mushrooms, sliced
1 16-ounce can tomatoes, with liquid
1/2 cup beef broth
salt and pepper to taste
1/2 cup non-fat plain yogurt

Mix together flour and paprika and coat beef. Heat
oil in large non-stick frying pan and brown cubes of
beef a few at a time. Remove and keep warm. Stir in
pepper and onion. Then add all remaining ingredients except yogurt. Heat to boiling. Reduce heat to
low. Cover and simmer for 1 hour and 45 minutes,
or until beef is tender. Stir in yogurt before serving.

Beef Stroganoff (see pages 123, 124, 173, 174)

Serves 4
Calories per portion: 335
Preparation and cooking time: 20 minutes

1 tablespoon olive oil or butter
1 medium onion, finely chopped
1/2 pound button mushrooms, sliced
1 tablespoon flour
pinch ground red pepper
1 pound beef tenderloin fillet or rump, very
thinly sliced into bite-sized pieces
2 tablespoons dry sherry
3/4 cup beef broth
4 ounces reduced-fat sour cream
salt, if necessary

Heat oil in large non-stick frying pan and fry onion
until soft and just turning golden. Add mushrooms
and stir-fry over medium-high heat for 1 or 2 minutes. Combine flour and red pepper and toss with
beef. Add beef, tossed, to frying pan and stir-fry for
3 to 4 minutes. Add sherry and cook for 1 minute.
Add broth and cook for 1 minute; finally, add sour
cream. Warm through, correct seasoning, and serve.

Beef Stir-Fry (see pages 117, 173)

Serves 4
Calories per portion: 300
Preparation and cooking time: 20 minutes

1 tablespoon olive oil
3/4 pound rump steak, cut into thin strips
1 cup mushrooms, sliced
1 8-ounce can whole-kernel corn
8 scallions, chopped
1 sweet red pepper, sliced
1 tablespoon sherry
2 teaspoons honey
pinch ground ginger
1 tablespoon soy sauce
1 tablespoon cornstarch mixed with 4 tablespoons water

In large non-stick frying pan or wok, heat oil and
stir-fry beef for 1 or 2 minutes over high heat, until
browned. Add vegetables and stir-fry for another 2
minutes. Add sherry and honey and stir. Finally,
add ginger, soy sauce, and cornstarch mixture. Heat
to a boil and thicken. Serve.

Sweet-and-Sour Pork (see pages 134, 145, 171, 174)

Serves 4
Calories per portion: 300
Preparation and cooking time: 1 hour and 5
minutes

1 tablespoon olive oil
1 pound loin of pork, cubed
1¾ cups chicken broth
salt and pepper to taste
1 sweet red pepper, sliced
1 sweet green pepper, sliced
1 8-ounce can pineapple chunks in natural
juice or water
1 tablespoon soy sauce
2 tablespoons soft brown sugar
2 tablespoons vinegar
1 tablespoon cornstarch

Heat oil in flameproof casserole and brown pork.
Add stock and seasoning. Place in oven at 300° F. for
1 hour. Return casserole dish to stove top. Add peppers and pineapple and simmer for a few minutes.
Mix together soy sauce, sugar, vinegar, and cornstarch. Add mixture to casserole. Stir until sauce
thickens and bubbles. Serve.

Pork Chops with Rosemary (see page 171)

Serves 4
Calories per serving 200
Preparation and cooking time: 25 minutes

4 loin pork chops
1 tablespoon onion, minced
1 garlic clove, minced
1 teaspoon rosemary leaves, dried, crumbled
1/3 cup dry red wine or chicken broth
salt and pepper to taste

Trim all fat from chops. In non-stick skillet, over medium heat, brown chops on all sides. Add onion, garlic, rosemary, and wine. Heat to boiling. Reduce heat to low, cover, and simmer 10 to 15 minutes, or until chops are fork-tender. Remove chops to serving platter. Boil sauce 3 minutes to thicken slightly. Season with salt and pepper and pour over chops. Serve.

Marinated Ginger Pork (see pages 118, 138)

Serves 4
Calories per serving: 300
Preparation and cooking time: 30 minutes
Marinating time: 4 hours

1/2 cup soy sauce
1-inch piece fresh ginger, peeled and minced
1 garlic clove, minced
1 pound pork tenderloin, whole

In large sealable plastic bag combine all ingredients. Seal and refrigerate 4 hours or overnight. Broil or grill meat 6 inches from heat or flame about 20 minutes or just until meat is no longer pink. Slice and serve.

GRINDING IT OUT
The Making of McDonald's
by
RAY KROC
with Robert Anderson

Few entrepreneurs can claim to have actually changed the way we live, but Ray Kroc was one of them. His revolutionary approach to fast-food service has earned him a place among the men who founded not merely businesses but new ways of living.

Not your typical self-made tycoon, Kroc was 52 when he met the McDonald brothers and opened his first franchise. Twenty-five years later, Kroc found himself in charge of the most successful and widespread fast-food operation the world had ever seen.

Now, in his own words, Ray Kroc will tell you the story of his incredible road to success. Irrepressible enthusiast and perceptive people-watcher, his stories will fascinate and inspire you.

"COLUMBUS DISCOVERED AMERICA, JEFFERSON INVENTED IT, AND RAY KROC BIG MAC'D IT."
—Tom Robbins, *Esquire* magazine

COOKING? DIETING? HERE'S HELP!

THE FOOD ALLERGY COOKBOOK
Allergy Information Association
_____ 90185-2 $4.95 U.S.

EASY, SWEET AND SUGARFREE
Karen E. Barkie
_____ 90282-4 $3.50 U.S.   _____ 90283-2 $4.50 Can.

BLOOMINGDALE'S EAT HEALTHY DIET
Laura Stein
_____ 90641-2 $3.95 U.S.   _____ 90642-0 $4.95 Can.

MARY ELLEN'S HELP YOURSELF DIET PLAN
Mary Ellen Pinkham
_____ 90237-9 $2.95 U.S.   _____ 90238-7 $3.95 Can.

THE BOOK OF WHOLE GRAINS
Marlene Anne Bumgarner
_____ 90072-4 $4.95 U.S.   _____ 90073-2 $6.25 Can.

Publishers Book and Audio Mailing Service
P.O. Box 120159, Staten Island, NY 10312-0004

Please send me the book(s) I have checked above. I am enclosing
$ _____ (please add $1.25 for the first book, and $.25 for each
additional book to cover postage and handling. Send check or
money order only—no CODs.)

Name _____

Address _____

City _____ State/Zip _____

Please allow six weeks for delivery. Prices subject to change
without notice.